MASTERING BIPOLAR DISORDER

Your Stress-Free Roadmap to Understanding, Coping, and Achieving Mental Stability

JASON L. BROWN

Copyright © 2024 Jason L. Brown. All rights reserved.

The content within this book may not be reproduced, duplicated, or transmitted without direct written permission from the author or the publisher.

Under no circumstances will any blame or legal responsibility be held against the publisher, or author, for any damages, reparation, or monetary loss due to the information contained within this book, either directly or indirectly.

Legal Notice:

This book is copyright protected. It is only for personal use. You cannot amend, distribute, sell, use, quote, or paraphrase any part of the content within this book, without the consent of the author or publisher.

Disclaimer Notice:

Please note the information contained within this document is for educational and entertainment purposes only. All effort has been expended to present accurate, up-to-date, reliable, and complete information. No warranties of any kind are declared or implied. Readers acknowledge that the author is not engaged in the rendering of legal, financial, medical, or professional advice. The content within this book has been derived from various sources. Please consult a licensed professional before attempting any techniques outlined in this book.

By reading this document, the reader agrees that under no circumstances is the author responsible for any losses, direct or indirect, that are incurred as a result of the use of the information contained within this document, including, but not limited to, errors, omissions, or inaccuracies.

CONTENTS

Introduction	7
1. UNDERSTANDING BIPOLAR DISORDER	9
Decoding Bipolar Disorder: Types and Symptoms	10
The Science behind Bipolar Disorder: What Happens in the Brain?	12
Bipolar I vs. Bipolar II: A Detailed Comparison	13
Recognizing Early Warning Signs and Triggers	16
The Role of Genetics and Environment in Bipolar Disorder	17
Debunking Myths: What Bipolar Disorder Is Not	19
2. DAILY MANAGEMENT STRATEGIES	23
Structuring Your Day for Mood Stability	23
Nutrition and Exercise: Their Impact on Bipolar Disorder	25
Sleep Hygiene Practices to Manage Mood Swings	26
The Importance of Routine in Bipolar Management	28
Stress Reduction Techniques That Work	30
Harnessing Creativity and Hobbies for Emotional Balance	32
3. MEDICATION AND TREATMENT OPTIONS	35
Overview of Medication Options: What You Need to Know	35
Psychotherapy and Bipolar Disorder: Finding the Right Fit	37
New Frontiers: Latest Research and Innovative Treatments	40
Managing Side Effects and Medication Interactions	42
The Role of Holistic Therapies in Treatment Plans	44
When to Consider Hospitalization: Guidance and Preparation	46

4. SUPPORT SYSTEMS AND RELATIONSHIPS ... 51
   Building a Reliable Support Network ... 51
   Communication Strategies for Discussing Bipolar Disorder ... 53
   How Partners Can Support During Mood Episodes ... 55
   Navigating Bipolar Disorder with Children in the Family ... 57
   Workplace Dynamics: Advocating for Yourself Professionally ... 59
   Finding and Utilizing Support Groups and Online Resources ... 61

5. COPING MECHANISMS AND RESILIENCE BUILDING ... 67
   Cognitive Behavioral Techniques for Mood Management ... 67
   Mindfulness and Meditation: Practices for Focus and Calm ... 69
   The Role of Journaling in Emotional Clarity ... 71
   Developing Personal Crisis Management Plans ... 73
   Overcoming Negative Thought Patterns ... 75
   Celebrating Small Wins: Building Blocks of Resilience ... 77

6. SPECIAL CONSIDERATIONS IN BIPOLAR DISORDER ... 81
   Bipolar Disorder in Women: Pregnancy and Hormonal Effects ... 81
   The Impact of Aging on Bipolar Disorder ... 83
   Substance Use and Bipolar Disorder: Navigating Dual Diagnosis ... 85
   Seasonal Affective Disorder and Bipolar: Managing Seasonal Changes ... 87
   Bipolar Disorder and Co-existing Health Conditions ... 89
   Legal Considerations: Rights and Responsibilities ... 91

7. EMPOWERMENT THROUGH EDUCATION ... 95
   Understanding Your Rights as a Patient ... 95
   Educating Friends and Family: Workshops and Resources ... 98
   Accessing and Interacting with Medical Research ... 100
   The Importance of Ongoing Education in Managing Bipolar Disorder ... 102

Leveraging Technology for Health Tracking and Management	104
Preparing for Doctor Visits and Therapy Sessions	106
8. LIVING A FULFILLING LIFE WITH BIPOLAR DISORDER	**109**
Success Stories: Real-Life Examples of Overcoming Challenges	109
Maintaining Long-Term Relationships While Managing Bipolar Disorder	111
Career Planning and Progression with Bipolar Disorder	114
Long-Term Financial Planning and Stability	116
Travel and Leisure: Enjoying Life Responsibly	118
Setting and Achieving Personal Goals Despite Bipolar Disorder	120
Conclusion	125
References	129

INTRODUCTION

Seeking a balance between the waves of euphoria and despair that come with bipolar is challenging. However, the true struggle is navigating the world's misunderstandings. Five years ago, during a moment of balance, I sat in the stillness of a doctor's office, absorbing my diagnosis. It was a pivotal turning point that reshaped my understanding of myself and my vision of what life could be. This book springs from that moment of clarity and the experiences that followed, marked by challenges, learnings, and unexpected gifts.

The purpose of this book is simple yet ambitious: to demystify bipolar disorder. It is crafted for you—whether you are grappling with the condition yourself, caring for someone who is, or simply seeking to understand this intricate aspect of human psychology. Here, you will find a blend of personal insights, professional knowledge, and the latest research, all aimed at shedding light on effective management and coping strategies. This is more than just a guide; it is a companion.

I have a personal connection to bipolar disorder as I live with it every day. Diagnosed five years ago, I traversed the complex maze of treatments and emotions that accompany this condition. My experiences—both challenging and rewarding—fuel my passion to support others on this path. I am committed to advocating for better mental health awareness and providing practical, hopeful resources for those affected.

This book is structured to guide you through understanding the nuances of bipolar I and II, embracing effective daily management techniques, medication and therapy options, and harnessing the power of support groups. What sets this book apart is its holistic approach—it is about confronting the challenges and recognizing and cultivating the opportunities for personal growth, resilience, and joy that bipolar disorder presents. Each chapter builds on the next, creating a comprehensive roadmap that addresses not just the "what" and the "how" but also the "why," making it easier for you to follow and read what is relevant to you.

As you turn these pages, I invite you to keep an open mind and a hopeful heart. Engage with the stories, strategies, and studies shared here. See how they connect with you and your experiences. Let this book serve as your steadfast companion, offering tools and insights that can light your way forward.

You are not alone in this. With the right knowledge and support, stability and happiness are not just possible—they are within your reach. Together, let's explore the complexities of bipolar disorder and move toward a life marked by deeper understanding and sustained joy.

CHAPTER 1

UNDERSTANDING BIPOLAR DISORDER

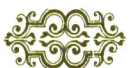

On a crisp autumn morning, a friend of mine named Sarah found herself buying plane tickets for a spontaneous trip around the world—a decision that felt exhilarating. Yet, three days later, she could not muster the energy to pack a suitcase or even get out of bed. This was not just a change of mind; it was a vivid illustration of the unpredictable swings of bipolar disorder. Sarah had been dealing with this since her diagnosis at twenty-two. The dramatic highs and lows of bipolar disorder make ordinary decisions difficult and emotional.

In this chapter, we will explore the complicated nature of bipolar disorder, a condition that affects millions yet remains shrouded in misunderstanding (National Institute of Mental Health, 2024). You will discover the distinct types of bipolar disorder, look into the symptoms, and understand how they impact daily life. We will also discuss the importance of an accurate diagnosis, which is crucial for effective management. Understanding these aspects of the disorder creates a foundation for success—whether you are dealing with the diagnosis yourself or supporting someone who is.

DECODING BIPOLAR DISORDER: TYPES AND SYMPTOMS

Bipolar disorder manifests in several forms, each with distinct characteristics and challenges. The primary types include Bipolar I, Bipolar II, and Cyclothymic Disorder. Bipolar I is often characterized by manic episodes that last at least seven days or are severe enough to require immediate hospital care. These episodes are contrasted by depressive periods lasting two weeks or more. Bipolar II involves a pattern of depressive episodes interspersed with hypomanic episodes. These episodes are similar to manic episodes but less severe and without the psychotic features often found in bipolar I. Cyclothymic Disorder, or Cyclothymia, involves periods of hypomanic symptoms interspersed with periods of depressive symptoms. While the fluctuation between highs and lows in Cyclothymia is often less intense, it can still significantly impact a person's life (National Institute of Mental Health, 2024).

Understanding the symptomatology of these types is crucial. Manic episodes can include feelings of euphoria, jumpiness, and increased self-importance, coupled with increased activity levels, rapid speech, decreased need for sleep, and sometimes reckless behavior. I know firsthand how these episodes can lead to significant disruptions in life, affecting everything from personal relationships to job stability. Hypomanic episodes share some of these characteristics. However, they are less likely to result in hospitalization or cause major impairment in work or social activities, like a manic episode (National Institute of Mental Health, 2024).

Depressive episodes, on the other hand, present with symptoms such as feeling intense sadness and anxiety, struggling to concentrate and complete even simple tasks, feelings of hopelessness, and a loss of interest in activities once enjoyed. You might even find that you talk slower and sleep too much (National Institute of

Mental Health, 2024). In my experience, the severity of these symptoms can lead to substantial difficulty in day-to-day functioning. The oscillation between these highs and lows can be confusing and exhausting for you and those around you, significantly impacting decision-making, relationships, and professional life.

I have personally found the symptoms manifest in a variety of ways. When I am manic, I struggle with impulse control, making decisions from an emotional place rather than a wise one. During depressive episodes, it is a push to get out of bed, let alone get to work and do my job with enthusiasm. Not even my favorite hobbies can get me excited. Everything feels harder. However, these symptoms can be controlled. The first step in finding balance is consulting with a medical professional and getting a diagnosis.

The challenge of diagnosing bipolar disorder lies in its complexity and the variability of its presentation. An accurate diagnosis, which often involves a physical exam, psychiatric assessment, and mood charting, is crucial for effective management. This process guarantees the treatment plan is tailored to your specific needs, enhancing the likelihood of managing the condition successfully (Mayo Clinic, n.d.).

Understanding bipolar disorder is the first step toward effective management. With a diagnosis and understanding of the disorder, you can make informed decisions about your health. It provides a framework for understanding the experiences and challenges that come with this condition. With knowledge comes the power to advocate for yourself and to seek out the resources and support that can help you lead a fulfilling life despite the ups and downs of bipolar disorder.

THE SCIENCE BEHIND BIPOLAR DISORDER: WHAT HAPPENS IN THE BRAIN?

Peering into the intricate workings of the brain during episodes of bipolar disorder can be as complex as understanding the disorder itself. However, the years of studies and research can offer some illumination on why those with bipolar disorder experience such extreme mood swings. There are a variety of causes, such as genetic and environmental causes. There is a neurological component to bipolar as well. At the core of bipolar-related fluctuations are neurobiological mechanisms, primarily involving neurotransmitter imbalances and notable changes in brain structure (Bressert, 2021).

Neurotransmitters, the brain's chemical messengers, play pivotal roles in regulating mood and behavior. In the context of bipolar disorder, key neurotransmitters such as serotonin, dopamine, and norepinephrine are often out of balance. This neurotransmitter imbalance disrupts the brain's usual signaling pathways, leading to the symptoms observed in bipolar disorder (Bressert, 2021).

The structural changes in the brains of individuals with bipolar disorder also provide insights into the condition's complexities. Studies have shown differences in the volume of certain brain regions that regulate mood and memory. For example, the hippocampus, a part of the brain responsible for mood and impulse control, often shows abnormalities in those with bipolar disorder. These structural anomalies offer insight into the progression of the illness and the emotional and cognitive challenges that are characteristic of the disorder (Bressert, 2021).

Advancements in neuroimaging, such as Magnetic Resonance Imaging (MRI) and Positron Emission Tomography (PET) scans, have revolutionized our understanding of bipolar disorder. These technologies have helped researchers find associations between brain markers derived from the MRI and bipolar disorder (Kohshour et al., 2022). PET scans have been used to measure activity in a resting state (Keener and Phillips, 2007). Such insights are invaluable for diagnosing bipolar disorder more accurately and tailoring more effective treatments.

Moreover, exploring how bipolar disorder relates to other neurological and psychiatric conditions deepens our understanding and diagnostic precision. Conditions such as anxiety, post-traumatic stress disorder (PTSD), and attention deficit hyperactivity disorder (ADHD) are commonly experienced among people with bipolar disorder. It is also not uncommon for people to have an eating disorder or substance abuse disorder as well (Bressert, 2021).

Research continues to peel back layers of complexity in the brain functions associated with bipolar disorder. These studies deepen our understanding and challenge us to rethink how we approach treatment. They bridge the gap between experiencing symptoms and recognizing them as part of a broader neurological pattern. This knowledge empowers patients and caregivers to visualize bipolar disorder as a series of emotional extremes and a manageable condition with identifiable, science-based origins.

BIPOLAR I VS. BIPOLAR II: A DETAILED COMPARISON

Understanding the nuances between Bipolar I and Bipolar II is crucial for accurate diagnosis and effective management. While both types fall under the umbrella of bipolar disorder, their diagnostic criteria, as in the Diagnostic and Statistical Manual (DSM-5), highlight significant differences primarily in the severity and duration of manic or hypomanic episodes.

Bipolar I disorder is characterized by manic episodes that may be preceded or followed by hypomanic or major depressive episodes. Bipolar II disorder is defined by a pattern of one or more major depressive episodes accompanied by at least one hypomanic episode without ever reaching the full criteria for a manic episode (Harrell, 2020).

These distinctions are not merely clinical; they translate into varied experiences in daily life and require different approaches to treatment. For individuals with Bipolar I, the presence of full-blown manic episodes can lead to more severe disruptions. Manic episodes might involve pleasurable feelings as you feel full of excitement and confidence. However, it is possible for mania to escalate into unwanted, destructive, and impulsive behaviors (Tartakovsky, 2021). Meanwhile, those with Bipolar II might not experience the highs as intensely, but the frequent and sometimes prolonged periods of depression can deeply affect their quality of life, making it challenging to maintain steady eating, sleeping, and socializing (Stanborough, 2022).

The impact on lifestyle and stress management is also distinctly different between the two types. Individuals with Bipolar I may find it more important to carefully plan travel and special events because they are potential mania triggers (Tartovsky, 2021). In contrast, those with Bipolar II may struggle more with doing things they know they need to do, which can make daily tasks and self-care overwhelming (Stanborough, 2022). I have found social interactions for Bipolar I individuals can be strained during manic phases due to impulsivity and grandiosity, whereas those with Bipolar II might withdraw socially during depressive phases, finding it hard to connect with others even when they desire to do so.

When it comes to treatment, the approaches need to be as tailored as the experiences of those living with each type. For Bipolar I, mood stabilizers are often the cornerstone of treatment to help control the ups and downs. Antipsychotic medications may also be used, especially if severe agitation is present (Lee and Swartz, n.d.). In contrast, the treatment regimen for Bipolar II may rely more heavily on a combination of antidepressants and mood stabilizers to manage the depressive episodes. Psychotherapy plays a critical role in both types but might focus on different aspects; for example, Bipolar I therapy might focus on effectively managing stress and triggers for manic episodes, while Bipolar II therapy might focus more on developing strategies to help cope with symptoms (Fletcher, 2023).

Consider the hypothetical scenario of John and Lisa, where John has Bipolar I, and Lisa has Bipolar II. John's condition might lead him to make impulsive decisions like investing all his savings into a risky business venture during a manic episode. Periods of severe depression may follow, where he struggles to face the repercussions of his actions. Lisa might consistently struggle with feelings of inadequacy and prolonged depressive states that make it difficult for her to seek out or maintain employment despite having periods of heightened productivity during hypomanic episodes. Their daily lives, challenges, and the support they require from loved ones vary significantly, illustrating why personalized treatment and understanding are key to managing their distinct conditions effectively.

This understanding of Bipolar I and II aids in better management and increased empathy toward those affected. Recognizing the specific challenges faced by individuals with either type of bipolar disorder allows caregivers, family members, and healthcare providers to offer the right support at the right time, tailored to the unique needs of the individual. As we continue to learn from each person's experience with bipolar disorder, our strategies for support, intervention, and care will only become more effective.

RECOGNIZING EARLY WARNING SIGNS AND TRIGGERS

In managing bipolar disorder, one of the most empowering tools at your disposal is the ability to recognize early warning signs of both manic and depressive episodes. This awareness is crucial for you and those who play a supportive role in helping manage these episodes effectively.

Early signs of a manic episode can include a noticeable increase in activity levels, reduced need for sleep, unusually elevated mood or irritability, rapid speech, racing thoughts, and sometimes grandiose ideas or overconfidence. Warning signs of a depressive episode might include feelings of sadness or unexplained crying spells, significant changes in appetite or sleep patterns, feelings of worthlessness, difficulty concentrating, and withdrawal from activities that were once enjoyed (National Institute of Mental Health, 2024).

The role of self-monitoring cannot be overstressed in managing bipolar disorder. By recognizing your triggers and tracking your moods and sleep, you can potentially see oncoming episodes. Tools such as journaling are invaluable in this regard, providing a structured way to monitor your well-being. This mindfulness helps in recognizing early signs. It also assists in communicating effectively with healthcare providers about your condition, leading to timely and appropriate interventions (Casabianca, 2021).

Environmental and emotional triggers play a significant role in the onset of bipolar episodes. Common triggers include stress, whether from emotionally charged personal relationships, work pressures, or "good" stress like moving to a new home or getting a job. Sleep disturbances can also precipitate manic or depressive episodes. Even climate and weather changes can trigger mood episodes (Gillette, 2023). Understanding what triggers your episodes is a critical step in managing them. This might require you to become a keen observer of your environments and interactions, noting what circumstances or stressors precipitate changes in your mood or behavior.

Once you identify these triggers, you can implement preventive strategies to minimize their impact. Stress management plans include relaxation techniques and healthy communication strategies. Structuring your day to include sufficient rest can also help in stabilizing your mood. Making lifestyle modifications like avoiding alcohol and recreational drugs. In some cases, it may be necessary to work with a therapist to develop strategies for coping with stress and emotional upheaval more constructively (Gillette, 2023).

By integrating these strategies into your daily life, you equip yourself with the tools to cope with bipolar disorder, allowing you to thrive. Recognizing early signs and understanding triggers allows for a proactive approach to managing your condition, one that emphasizes your strength and capacity for resilience.

THE ROLE OF GENETICS AND ENVIRONMENT IN BIPOLAR DISORDER

Our genetic makeup and the environments we live in play a significant role in the expression of bipolar disorder. Understanding this is about uncovering the condition's roots and forging pathways toward more effective prevention and personalized treatment strategies. Let's explore how these elements intertwine in the context of bipolar disorder, shedding light on why some individuals develop the condition while others do not, despite similar genetic predispositions.

Bipolar disorder, like many mental health conditions, does not follow a simple pattern of inheritance. Research indicates that 70-80% of individuals with bipolar disorder can be attributed to genetic factors (Fabbri, 2021). The exact genetic paths can be complex. Studies suggest that multiple genes, each contributing a small effect, combine to increase the risk of developing the disorder. This polygenic nature means that no single gene causes the disorder; rather, multiple genes interact to create a significant risk. Ongoing genetic research continues to explore these relationships. These studies are crucial, helping to identify potential genetic markers that could be targeted in future treatments or used to predict the onset of the condition more accurately (Pederson, 2021).

However, genetics only tells part of the story. Environmental factors play a critical role in the manifestation and management of bipolar disorder. For example, the presence of trauma in early life and the amount of emotional support people receive can significantly influence whether and how bipolar disorder manifests. Life events such as financial crises and work-related challenges trigger the onset of bipolar disorder in genetically predisposed individuals (Aldinger and Schulze, 2017).

The gene-environment interaction model provides a useful framework for understanding how genetics and environmental factors combine to influence the development of bipolar disorder. This model suggests that while genetic predispositions set the stage, environmental factors act as catalysts that can either trigger the condition or influence its course (Quinn and D'Onofrio, 2020). For example, a person might carry genetic variations that increase their vulnerability to bipolar disorder. Whether they develop the condition might depend on a complex mix of factors such as stress levels, social support, and exposure to trauma. Conversely, someone with a similar genetic makeup in a supportive, low-stress environment might not develop the condition. This interaction emphasizes the importance of considering both genetic and environmental factors when diagnosing and treating bipolar disorder.

Understanding these genetic and environmental influences has profound implications for prevention and treatment. Knowing that a person has a higher genetic risk for bipolar disorder can lead to earlier monitoring and intervention, potentially staving off the onset or reducing the severity of the condition. Interventions focusing on modifying environmental factors—such as maintaining a regular schedule, reducing stress through therapy or other means, and building robust support networks—can significantly impact the management of the disorder. These plans might include tailored pharmacological combined with psychotherapeutic approaches (Lebow, 2022).

As we continue to uncover more about the genetic underpinnings and environmental influences, our ability to intervene effectively and help individuals lead stable, fulfilling lives develops. This ongoing path of discovery challenges us to rethink our approaches to mental health. It also offers hope through personalized understanding and intervention. We can significantly improve the quality of life for those affected by bipolar disorder as we develop an understanding of the disorder.

DEBUNKING MYTHS: WHAT BIPOLAR DISORDER IS NOT

Some of the most significant barriers to understanding and effectively managing bipolar disorder are misconceptions and myths that surround it. These myths distort public perception. They contribute to the stigma that many individuals with the disorder face daily. It is crucial to address and debunk these myths head-on.

A common myth is that bipolar disorder is the same for anyone with the disorder. This misconception minimizes the seriousness of the disorder and can prevent individuals from seeking individualized professional help. Everyone's experience with bipolar disorder is different. For some, they experience episodes of severe depression followed by manic episodes resulting in increased energy. Others may experience hypomanic episodes, which cause symptoms less severe than those of a manic episode. Triggers and responses may vary from person to person as well, impacting their lives differently (Grey, 2024).

Another damaging myth is the belief that bipolar disorder is a sign of weak character or a lack of willpower and that people with bipolar disorder cannot thrive at work or in school. This stigma is hurtful and unfounded. Bipolar disorder is a medical condition linked to biological changes in the brain, and it requires understanding and medical treatment, not judgment. While bipolar disorder can certainly affect these areas, it is also possible to thrive. With the right treatment and assistance from a medical professional, symptoms can be managed, allowing individuals to succeed (Grey, 2024).

In distinguishing bipolar disorder from other mental health issues, it is crucial to recognize that while there are overlapping symptoms, each condition has unique characteristics and treatment approaches. For instance, while major depressive disorder involves significant depressive episodes, it lacks the manic or hypomanic episodes characteristic of bipolar disorder (Borenstein, 2020). Similarly, while personality disorders may involve mood swings, with behavioral disorders like borderline personality disorder, impulsive urges may occur anytime, but for bipolar patients, they are typically tied to manic episodes (Ferguson, 2021). Schizophrenia, while also involving mood disturbances like hallucinations and delusions, might not be present in bipolar disorder unless during severe manic or depressive episodes (Ginta, 2022). Clarifying these distinctions is not just a matter of semantics; it is essential for diagnosis, treatment, and the understanding of what individuals with each condition experience.

The impact of misinformation on the perception of bipolar disorder in society is profound. Stereotypes and sensationalized portrayals in media can lead to difficulties within relationships, lower self-esteem, and a lack of hope. This stigma can prevent individuals from seeking help for symptoms out of fear of being labeled or judged, potentially leading to worse outcomes in their personal and professional lives (American Psychiatric Association, n.d.).

Education plays a pivotal role in transforming societal attitudes and improving the lives of those affected by bipolar disorder. By promoting a better understanding of the condition through accurate information, we can cultivate empathy, reduce stigma, and encourage a more supportive environment for those affected. Each step taken toward education and understanding represents progress toward a society that supports rather than stigmatizes, providing those with bipolar disorder a better chance at a full and rewarding life (American Psychiatric Association, n.d.).

Through these efforts, we challenge old myths and change how society views bipolar disorder, empowering those affected to seek help confidently, manage their symptoms effectively, and advocate for their needs. Changing perceptions is a long process and requires the commitment of individuals, communities, and institutions. Each conversation that corrects a misconception, each story that sheds light on the reality of living with bipolar disorder, and each piece of educational material that replaces ignorance with insight adds up to a more understanding and compassionate world.

CHAPTER 2

DAILY MANAGEMENT
STRATEGIES

Life with bipolar disorder is marked by highs and lows, punctuated by periods of balance. Managing your day effectively is like strategically painting over the chaos with structured routines and mindful practices. It can transform this canvas into a masterpiece of stability and color.

STRUCTURING YOUR DAY FOR MOOD STABILITY

For someone living with bipolar disorder, a schedule can help them manage the disorder. This balance is crucial. It involves bringing together work, rest, and leisure in a way that does not trigger the disorder. Consider what should be included in the routine. Things like taking prescribed medication, carefully planning for enough sleep, and establishing a structure that works (Currin-Sheehan, 2021).

The importance of consistent timing in your daily routine cannot be overstated. It serves as the backbone of mood stability, helping with worry and anxiety. By waking up and sleeping at the same times each day, you create a rhythm that your body and mind can rely on, reducing the likelihood of mood fluctuations. This consistency creates a sense of normalcy and control (McMillen, 2021).

Effective time management is another crucial aspect of structuring your day. It involves prioritizing tasks based on urgency and your personal energy fluctuations throughout the day. Start by identifying your top priorities for the day and allocate specific times to focus on these tasks or block them into your calendar. Use tools like planners or digital apps to keep track of tasks and deadlines, breaking larger projects into smaller, manageable steps. Do not forget something as simple as taking a short break to enjoy a cup of tea after completing a task will help you stay motivated and productive (Martins, 2024).

However, while structure is beneficial, it is equally important to maintain flexibility in your routines to accommodate mood fluctuations. For instance, if you wake up feeling low, you might choose to shift your schedule around to prioritize unstructured time when you can meditate and find your happy place. This adaptive approach empowers you to respond to your body's needs while still maintaining a sense of structure and productivity. It is about finding the balance between rigidity and chaos—structuring your day enough to provide stability but also allowing room for adjustments as needed (Currin-Sheehan, 2021).

By mastering the art of structuring your day, you cultivate stability and reclaim the power to shape your daily experiences. This proactive stance on managing your time and activities serves as a fundamental step toward achieving balance. Embrace these strategies with patience and persistence, and watch as your days transform into a harmonious blend of productivity and peace, mirroring the stability you seek.

NUTRITION AND EXERCISE: THEIR IMPACT ON BIPOLAR DISORDER

When you start on the path to managing bipolar disorder, you are often confronted with the challenge of balancing medication and therapy. However, lifestyle challenges like nutrition and exercise can make a difference. These elements of daily living exert a profound influence on mood stability and can serve as foundational components of your holistic management plan.

Nutrition plays a critical role in brain health, and certain nutrients have been found to be particularly beneficial for those with bipolar disorder. Omega-3 fatty acids, for instance, are known for their ability to support brain function. Research suggests that they can play a role in smoothing out mood swings and are particularly effective in managing depressive symptoms. Foods rich in omega-3s, such as salmon, flaxseeds, and eggs, should be a staple in your diet (Krans, 2024). Similarly, B vitamins, especially B1 and B12, are great in easing anxiety and irritability as well as providing energy (Currin-Sheehan and Martin, 2021). Sticking to a diet that maintains these essential nutrient levels can help manage bipolar disorder (Krans, 2024).

The overall balance of nutrients also matters significantly. In my experience, planning meals can seem daunting, but starting with simple changes like incorporating a variety of fruits, vegetables, whole grains, and protein sources is a great way to start. Consider preparing balanced meals that sustain your energy levels and stabilize your mood. If meal planning is overwhelming, simple tools like meal planning apps or a consultation with a nutritionist can provide structured support.

The benefits of exercise extend beyond physical health, especially for those managing bipolar disorder. Regular physical activity can have a potent effect on mood. Engaging in exercise leads to the release of endorphins, often known as 'feel-good' hormones, which can naturally lift your mood and reduce feelings of depression. Moreover, exercise aids in stress reduction, another crucial aspect of managing bipolar disorder. As we have discussed, stress is a common trigger for mood episodes, and finding natural, effective ways to reduce stress is paramount (Wells, 2019).

The type of exercise you choose can be adapted to how you are feeling on any given day. Over time, I have found certain exercises to be more helpful in certain moods. During depressive phases, when energy may be low, gentle activities like yoga or walking can be particularly beneficial. These activities can significantly boost mood and energy levels. On days when you feel more energetic or are experiencing hypomanic symptoms, channeling that energy into more intense aerobic exercises like running or cycling can be beneficial. These activities can help in using up the excess energy in a productive way, potentially easing the intensity of hypomanic episodes.

Incorporating regular exercise into your routine does not have to be a chore or another stressor. It can be as simple as a daily fifteen-minute walk, gradually increasing the time as you feel more comfortable. The key is consistency and listening to your body. Over time, regular physical activity boosts your physical health, becoming a crucial part of managing your mood and enhancing your overall quality of life. When incorporated alongside a healthy and nutritious diet, they can effectively help you manage your bipolar.

SLEEP HYGIENE PRACTICES TO MANAGE MOOD SWINGS

A restful night's sleep can be rejuvenating. For those managing bipolar disorder, the quality and quantity of sleep refreshes you and plays a pivotal role in mood regulation. Disturbances in sleep patterns can precipitate manic or depressive episodes, whereas balanced sleep can significantly mitigate these risks (Purse, 2023).

Understanding the connection between sleep and mood regulation is crucial. Sleep deprivation can potentially trigger manic episodes. A disturbance to your circadian rhythm can indicate a depressive phase. This bidirectional relationship means mood states affect sleep patterns, which can also profoundly influence mood states. Thus, maintaining a regulated sleep schedule is vital in managing the ebbs and flows of bipolar disorder effectively (Purse, 2023).

Developing a consistent sleep routine is instrumental in enhancing sleep quality. This routine starts with setting a fixed bedtime and wake-up time, even on weekends (Purse, 2023). As bedtime approaches, reducing exposure to blue light emitted by screens can help signal to your brain that it is time to wind down. You might consider establishing a nightly ritual that promotes relaxation, such as reading a book, taking a warm bath, or practicing gentle yoga stretches. These activities cue your body for sleep. They create a buffer zone between the day's stresses and nighttime rest, encouraging a tranquil transition into sleep (Suni, 2023).

Handling sleep disturbances efficiently is key to maintaining mood stability. Individuals with bipolar disorder often experience insomnia during manic phases (Purse, 2023). Addressing insomnia might involve creating a sleep routine, as we discussed earlier. On the other hand, dealing with hypersomnia—excessive sleepiness— requires a proactive approach to regulating sleep patterns. This might include exercising regularly and making sure you have a good sleep schedule (Morales-Brown, 2023).

The cautious use of sleep aids can also play a role in managing sleep issues, though they should always be approached with care and under medical supervision. While prescription sleep medications can provide short-term relief for sleep disturbances, they are not the only option. Natural alternatives, such as melatonin supplements or herbal teas like valerian root, can be effective in promoting sleep without the risks associated with prescription drugs. However, it is essential to consult with a healthcare provider before starting any new supplement, especially when managing a condition as complex as bipolar disorder (Mayo Clinic, n.d.).

Incorporating these sleep hygiene practices into your daily routine can significantly expand your ability to manage bipolar disorder. By prioritizing quality sleep, you equip your body with the resilience to handle mood fluctuations more effectively, paving the way for more stable and fulfilling days. As you continue to explore and implement these strategies, remember that small steps can lead to significant improvements in both your sleep and overall well-being.

THE IMPORTANCE OF ROUTINE IN BIPOLAR MANAGEMENT

Creating a routine provides a sense of healthy control and stability necessary to manage bipolar disorder. You will find stability in your routine, tailoring it to fit your specific needs and allowing for enough flexibility to respond appropriately to changes in mood.

A well-structured routine is a crucial part of managing bipolar disorder. It provides the stability and predictability that are essential in the daily lives of those affected. This stability helps to manage anxiety and significantly reduces the likelihood of severe mood swings. A well-planned routine offers you support, guiding your daily actions and helping stabilize your mood against the unpredictable elements of bipolar disorder (Currin-Sheehan, 2021).

Developing personalized routines that cater to individual needs, energy levels, and life commitments is not just beneficial; it is necessary. Aligning challenging tasks with high-energy times and more contemplative or relaxing activities with lower-energy times maximizes your effectiveness and maintains your mood balance (Mosunic, n.d.). For instance, if you are a morning person, you might schedule important meetings or demanding creative work during these hours and reserve afternoons for follow-ups or routine tasks that require less mental exertion.

Incorporating small, daily rituals into this routine can significantly heighten its effectiveness. Rituals act as anchors, providing moments of predictability and comfort that can greatly ease anxiety. These could be as simple as setting aside 10-15 minutes in the morning to enjoy a cup of coffee. These rituals become touchstones of normalcy and control amidst the flux of daily life and mood variability. They offer not just stability but also a sense of personal ritual that reinforces your autonomy over your day and, by extension, your emotional state (Plata, 2018).

I have found flexibility within the framework of stability allows you to respond to your needs without causing upheaval in your life. For example, if you begin to feel the onset of a depressive episode, you might choose to lighten your work schedule, allowing for more rest or engaging in therapeutic activities such as light exercise or art. Conversely, during a hypomanic episode, you might increase physical activities or channel your energy into structured creative projects to maintain balance. The key is to anticipate these changes and adapt your routine to suit your current state without losing the structure that provides overall stability. You can help yourself do this by tracking your mood to see how certain activities affect you (Gold, 2022).

This approach of personalized, flexible routine management can transform the way you live with bipolar disorder. It is about creating a life structure that supports your well-being consistently while also being adaptable enough to meet the changing needs dictated by your mood states. Embracing this strategy empowers you to take control of your disorder and live a life defined not by your condition but by your aspirations and achievements.

STRESS REDUCTION TECHNIQUES THAT WORK

Having a safe and healthy experience with bipolar disorder requires managing the symptoms and addressing the underlying stressors that can trigger mood episodes. When stress does hit, you can utilize relaxation techniques and certain behavioral strategies to cope with it. Building these into a stress management plan can properly prepare you to reduce and handle stress.

The first step in this process is identifying what these stressors are, which can often be as varied as the individuals experiencing them. Personal stressors might include relationship conflicts or financial worries, while environmental stressors could come from a stressful home or workplace. Recognizing these triggers is a crucial first step; this awareness allows you to develop strategies to mitigate their impact before they escalate into full-blown episodes (Vann, 2023).

Once you have identified your specific stressors, the next crucial step is learning effective techniques to manage your stress response. One powerful method is deep breathing exercises, which can quickly calm the mind and reduce anxiety. Techniques like "breath focus," where you take long, slow breaths and try to disengage from thoughts that distract or distress you, can be particularly effective in slowing down a racing heart and promoting relaxation.

Another method is body scanning, which involves tensing and then relaxing different muscle groups in your body. This combines progressive muscle relaxation and breath focus. This practice helps in reducing physical tension, aiding in diverting your focus away from stressors and grounding you in the present moment.

Mindfulness meditation offers substantial benefits in managing stress by seeking and reaching a state of awareness and presence. This practice involves observing your thoughts and feelings without judgment, which can be instrumental in changing your typical responses to stressful situations. By incorporating mindfulness into your daily routine, you can increase your resilience to stress and fortify your overall emotional and mental well-being (Harvard Health Publishing, 2022).

Beyond individual techniques, cognitive restructuring—a core component of cognitive-behavioral therapy (CBT)—is invaluable in changing stress-inducing thought patterns. This strategy involves identifying negative thoughts. Using Socratic Questioning, you can begin to challenge those negative thoughts and analyze them to see if they are true. Cognitive restructuring can help challenge problems, making stress more manageable and less likely to trigger a mood episode (Ackerman, 2018).

Creating a comprehensive stress management plan is like setting up a safety net to catch you when you inevitably encounter stressors. This plan might include daily practices such as the relaxation techniques mentioned, alongside strategies for self-care like taking breaks and listening to calming music (Mayo Clinic, n.d.). It is also important to recognize when professional help is needed. Understanding your limits and knowing when to seek support from a therapist or counselor can be crucial in preventing a minor stressor from causing a major setback in your management of bipolar disorder.

By integrating these stress reduction techniques into your life, you build a toolkit that helps in managing day-to-day stresses and your ability to plot a course for the challenges posed by bipolar disorder. Each technique is unique, and together, they can provide a robust defense against the potential upheavals triggered by stress. Engaging in these practices regularly can lead to significant improvements in your overall quality of life, empowering you to live more fully and with greater peace despite the challenges of bipolar disorder.

HARNESSING CREATIVITY AND HOBBIES FOR EMOTIONAL BALANCE

Engaging in creative activities offers more than just a way to fill time; it serves as a therapeutic outlet that can significantly enrich your emotional well-being. It is a wonderful form of creative expression. By integrating these practices into your daily routine, you can cope better, helping you manage your stress.

Creativity acts as a conduit for expressing yourself. This expression is particularly valuable in managing bipolar disorder, where emotions can often feel overwhelming or suppressed. Activities such as painting, writing, or playing music allow you to process these feelings in a constructive form that is healing. The act of creating something helps counteract feelings of worthlessness or frustration that may accompany depressive episodes (Cohut, 2018).

Consider the therapeutic power of hobbies like painting or gardening. These activities require a focus that can momentarily push aside persistent worries or intrusive thoughts, offering a mental break that can reduce stress levels. Engaging in a hands-on activity, like painting, can help release bottled-up anxiety. Gardening, on the other hand, encourages an optimistic attitude as you see the evidence of your hard work as the plants grow. The physical activity involved, combined with the nurturing aspect of caring for plants, can ground you in the present moment and lessen the grip of anxiety or agitation (Beasley, 2021).

Integrating these hobbies into your daily routine can elevate your well-being. This integration does not have to be overwhelming; it can be as simple as setting aside specific times in your week dedicated to your creative outlets. For instance, you might reserve Sunday afternoons for gardening or spend an hour each evening writing or sketching. The key is to make these activities as much a part of your routine as eating meals or taking medications. This regularity deepens your sense of self and adds depth and dimension to everyday life (Badosa, n.d.).

Using creativity as a coping tool helps manage stressful circumstances (Tahmaseb-McConatha, 2021). In my experience, I have found it helpful to adjust activities based on your mood. For example, during manic phases, channeling your heightened energy into creative projects can help regulate your mood. Activities that are immersive and demanding, like playing music or engaging in a complex craft, can harness this energy productively. In contrast, during depressive phases, simpler, more meditative artistic activities like coloring or playing slow, melodic songs on an instrument can provide solace and a sense of calm. The key is to align your creative activities with your current emotional state, using them as tools to restore balance and better your mood.

Creative expression offers a unique pathway to emotional balance, providing both an outlet and a distraction from the challenges of bipolar disorder. By regularly incorporating creative hobbies into your life, you enrich your days and build a repertoire of therapeutic tools that can support your stability. Engage with your creativity as a vital component of your wellness strategy, one that nourishes both your mind and spirit.

As we close this chapter on daily management strategies, we have explored how structured routines that include healthy nutrition and exercise, good sleep, and creative expression can help form a comprehensive toolkit for managing bipolar disorder. Each element contributes uniquely to stabilizing mood and enhancing quality of life, emphasizing the importance of a holistic approach to health. As you continue to apply these strategies, remember that each step forward, no matter how small, is a significant move toward stability and wellness. In the next chapter, we will learn more about understanding and exploring medication and treatment options, further equipping you with the knowledge to manage your condition effectively.

CHAPTER 3

MEDICATION AND TREATMENT OPTIONS

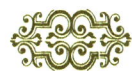

Managing bipolar disorder can be daunting. Sometimes, alternative methods are not enough to support you during manic, hypomanic, and depressive phases. If that's the case, it may be time to add some tools provided by a medical professional. This chapter is about equipping you with such tools, focusing here on the pharmacological therapies available for managing bipolar disorder—your medication options. This is your compass and map, guiding you through the complexities of treatment choices and how to use them effectively.

OVERVIEW OF MEDICATION OPTIONS: WHAT YOU NEED TO KNOW

Understanding bipolar disorder treatment begins with developing your knowledge of the different classes of medications typically prescribed. These are your mainstays: mood stabilizers, antipsychotics, and antidepressants, each serving a unique function in managing the disorder.

Mood stabilizers are the cornerstone of bipolar disorder treatment. They work by evening out the mood swings inherent to the condition. Other mood stabilizers include anticonvulsants. Each of these medications can help control or mitigate manic episodes (Cleveland Clinic, n.d.). Next in your arsenal are antipsychotics. These medications are effective in managing mood swings. These medications can be used in conjunction with mood stabilizers to help control symptoms, especially when they are acute or particularly disruptive (Meissner, 2024). Antidepressants are used cautiously in the treatment of bipolar disorder due to the risk they can pose in triggering manic episodes. However, when used in combination with a mood stabilizer or antipsychotic, antidepressants can be effective. The key here is careful management and monitoring, making sure they are used in a way that maximizes their benefit while minimizing risks (Nall, 2022).

The choice of medication, or combination of medications, depends on several factors. You will want to consider any potential side effects, other medications you may be taking, and pregnancy status. It is important to work alongside a medical professional to confirm the medications you are using are effective. Doctors can assist you during the trial-and-error process that comes with choosing medications. They are invaluable in managing side effects (Mayo Clinic, n.d.).

Finding the right medication is often a process that takes time. This experience can be frustrating, as it may take time to determine the most effective medication or combination of medications that work for you with manageable side effects. It typically starts with a thorough assessment of your symptoms. From there, your doctor might prescribe a medication, observing how you respond over a period of weeks or months. Adjustments—whether changing the dose, switching to a different medication, or adding another medication to your treatment plan—are often necessary based on your response and any side effects you experience (International Bipolar Foundation, n.d.).

The importance of medication adherence cannot be overstated. Sticking to your prescribed medication regime is crucial for its success. Non-adherence can lead to a relapse of symptoms, hospitalization, and, in some cases, can make the disorder more difficult to manage in the long run (Anderson, 2023). I have found setting daily reminders, using pill organizers, and integrating your medication regime into your daily routine to maintain consistency. Regular check-ins with your healthcare provider are also essential, providing an opportunity to discuss any challenges you are facing with your medication and to adjust as needed.

Medications are a key component in the management of bipolar disorder, offering a means to stabilize mood swings and develop a better quality of life. They must be used wisely and carefully, tailored to the individual's needs and conditions, addressing bipolar disorder safely and effectively. As you continue to explore these options, remember that patience and open communication with your healthcare provider are your best allies in this part of your treatment.

PSYCHOTHERAPY AND BIPOLAR DISORDER: FINDING THE RIGHT FIT

The complexities of bipolar disorder often require more than medication alone; psychotherapy plays an integral role in comprehensive treatment plans. The right type of psychotherapy can profoundly influence your management of bipolar disorder, offering tools and strategies that align with your specific needs and experiences. Once you have decided on a therapeutic approach, you will want to verify the method and therapist fit your needs. Psychotherapy, when combined with medication, can be a powerful tool for managing bipolar disorder. In fact, it can even benefit your loved ones. As we head into this chapter, Let's explore the different psychotherapeutic approaches that have been tailored to support individuals with bipolar disorder, including Cognitive Behavioral Therapy (CBT), Dialectical Behavior Therapy (DBT), and family-focused therapy.

Cognitive Behavioral Therapy (CBT) is a form of psychotherapy that helps you address problematic thoughts and behaviors. One of the core beliefs of CBT is that problems are based on, in part, problematic thinking and patterns of unhealthy behavior. CBT can help you challenge and reframe the negative thought patterns that often accompany depressive episodes, such as feelings of worthlessness or hopelessness. This approach aids in immediate symptom management. It equips you with lasting strategies to handle future challenges, potentially reducing the frequency and severity of mood swings (American Psychological Foundation, n.d.).

Dialectical Behavior Therapy (DBT) is a great tool for managing bipolar disorder due to its focus on teaching coping skills and enhancing emotional regulation. DBT emphasizes the development of four key skills: mindfulness, distress tolerance, emotion regulation, and interpersonal effectiveness (Psychology Today, n.d.). Family-focused therapy involves family members or caregivers in the therapeutic process, which is essential considering the significant impact bipolar disorder can have on personal relationships. This form of therapy educates family members about the disorder. It also equips them with strategies to communicate effectively during different phases of the disorder (Jarrold, 2023).

Choosing the appropriate type of therapy involves considering your specific symptoms, treatment goals, and personal preferences. For instance, if you find that your relationships are particularly strained by the emotional ups and downs of bipolar disorder, family-focused therapy might be beneficial. Alternatively, if you struggle with managing rapid mood changes or emotional crises, DBT might be a more suitable choice. There are many modes of therapy, even more than we have discussed. You are certain to find one that works for you. The decision should ideally be made in collaboration with a mental health professional who can assess your needs and recommend the most effective therapeutic approach based on their expertise (Nguyen, 2021).

Integrating therapy with medication forms the cornerstone of an effective bipolar disorder treatment plan. Mental health is complex and often requires multiple approaches to achieve maximum effectiveness. While medications can help stabilize mood swings chemically, psychotherapy addresses the behavioral and emotional aspects of the disorder, providing a safe space to address problems with a qualified therapist. This dual approach aims at symptom relief, developing a deeper understanding of your emotional patterns, and learning coping strategies that empower you to lead a more stable, fulfilling life. The convergence of these treatments expands their effectiveness, providing a more holistic approach to managing bipolar on a day-to-day basis. You are more likely to experience enhanced therapy outcomes when on the proper pharmaceutical treatment plan. The combination of both treatments helps create an individualized treatment plan (Ellie Mental Health, 2023).

For family members and caregivers, engaging in therapy themselves can be incredibly beneficial. It provides them with a deeper understanding of bipolar disorder, equipping them with the knowledge and tools to offer meaningful support and avoid perpetuating harmful stereotypes. Therapy sessions can serve as a safe space to express concerns and learn how to handle the emotional challenges that come with caring for someone with bipolar disorder, ultimately strengthening the support system around you (Substance Abuse and Mental Health Services Administration, 2019).

As you move forward, remember that the right therapeutic approach for you might change over time as your needs and circumstances change. Regularly discussing your progress with your therapist and being open to adjusting your treatment plan can help you stay on track and respond to changes in your condition effectively. Keep your mind open to trying new medications and modes of therapy, allowing yourself to find the treatment plan that manages your bipolar symptoms.

NEW FRONTIERS: LATEST RESEARCH AND INNOVATIVE TREATMENTS

With bipolar disorder treatment constantly developing, the horizon is continually brightened by new research and innovations that promise more personalized and effective care. New advancements in pharmaceuticals and therapy modes provide hope that you will find the combination that works best for you. As researchers develop a deeper understanding of the disorder and its genetic factors, more effective treatment plans are possible. In this section, we will discuss those advancements and their potential effect on bipolar disorder treatments.

One of the most exciting developments in recent years has been the advent of new and experimental medications that potentially offer greater efficacy and fewer side effects. These include drugs that modulate specific neurotransmitters or neural pathways that recent research has implicated in mood disorders. For example, researchers are exploring the potential of glutamate modulators, which could offer new hope for reducing what current medications sometimes fail to achieve. These novel treatments, still in the trial phase, are paving the way for what could be the next generation of psychiatric medication, potentially transforming lives with their approach and reduced side effects (Henter, Park, and Zarate, 2021).

Alongside these pharmacological advances, the integration of technology in bipolar disorder management has been groundbreaking. Digital mood trackers offer you and your healthcare provider real-time data on mood fluctuations, sleep patterns, and other triggers that can inform and refine your treatment plan. These tools enable a more dynamic response to the shifting sands of mood associated with bipolar disorder (NeuroLaunch, 2023). Telepsychiatry has also expanded dramatically, particularly highlighted by the global shift toward telehealth services during the COVID-19 pandemic. This technology guarantees you can access consistent and quality psychiatric care from the comfort of your home, reducing barriers to treatment such as transportation challenges or the stigma sometimes associated with visiting mental health clinics (Leonard, 2020).

The field of genetics and biomarker research is another area experiencing rapid growth, offering insights that could revolutionize how bipolar disorder is diagnosed and treated. Recent studies have identified genetic markers like AKAP11, which increases susceptibility to bipolar disorder, enhancing our understanding of the biological underpinnings of the condition (Eisenstadt, 2022). Biomarkers, characteristics that can be objectively measured to indicate normal biological processes, are also proving invaluable in predicting treatment outcomes. These help reduce the trial and error phase of treatment and correctly assess and diagnose conditions (Davies, 2020).

Looking to the future, the treatment of bipolar disorder seems poised to become increasingly personalized, moving beyond the one-size-fits-all approach. The integration of ongoing genetic research, innovative drug development, and advanced technologies promises a more nuanced understanding of the disorder and more precise treatment strategies. These developments are not just about managing symptoms but are aimed at fundamentally enhancing the quality of life for those affected by bipolar disorder, offering hope and a more stable path forward. This reduces stigma and promotes healing.

As these new frontiers in research and treatment continue to develop, there is a promise to improve care and challenge us to rethink our approaches to mental health disorders. The potential to customize treatments to the individual characteristics of each person's disorder represents a significant shift toward more effective and compassionate care.

MANAGING SIDE EFFECTS AND MEDICATION INTERACTIONS

When you begin a treatment plan for bipolar disorder that includes medication, understanding and managing side effects is crucial to maintaining your overall health and well-being. Medications such as mood stabilizers, antipsychotics, and antidepressants can bring much-needed relief, but they also come with their own set of challenges in the form of side effects. In this section, we will dive deeper into what these side effects may be, how medications might interact, and how making lifestyle adjustments and careful monitoring can help manage these side effects.

Navigating these side effects requires a combination of vigilance and proactive management. Some common side effects include nausea, weight gain, and drowsiness. For gastrointestinal upset, taking your medications with a meal may help with nausea. Weight gain, a common side effect, especially with some antipsychotic medications, can be managed through a balanced diet and regular physical activity. Adjusting the timing of your medication, such as taking sedative drugs closer to bedtime, can help mitigate their impact on your daily activities. Consulting with your healthcare provider is key, as they might adjust your dosage or suggest a different medication with fewer sedative effects (Meissner, 2021).

Another crucial aspect of managing your treatment effectively is understanding and avoiding potential drug interactions. Bipolar disorder medications can interact with various prescription and over-the-counter drugs, altering their effects and potentially increasing side effects. Certain prescription drug combinations can increase weight gain, interfere with the thyroid, and cause tremors (Osser, 2022). Always inform your healthcare provider about all the medications you are taking, including herbal supplements and over-the-counter drugs. This information helps your doctor to foresee potential adverse interactions and adjust your treatment plan accordingly.

Lifestyle adjustments play a significant role in minimizing side effects. Regular physical activity helps manage weight, boost mood, and combat fatigue. Being aware of your eating practices and verifying there are no interactions between the food and your medication is important. You can adjust your diet to reduce or increase specific foods as needed. You can make minor adjustments to your everyday life, improving the side effects you experience and your quality of life (MacMillan, 2022).

I have found regular monitoring and open communication with your healthcare provider to be essential. Keeping a detailed log of any side effects you experience—including when they occur, their intensity, and their impact on your daily life—provides valuable information that your healthcare provider can use to adjust your treatment plan. This log should be shared regularly with your doctor, who might adjust your medication dose, switch you to a different medication, or recommend additional treatments to manage side effects effectively. It is crucial to keep up honest and open communication with your doctor about the side effects you experience (U.S Food and Drug Administration, 2022).

In managing side effects and medication interactions, remember that your active participation and honest communication are key. Each person's experience with medication can vary significantly, so personalized adjustments are often necessary to find the most effective and comfortable treatment plan. Engaging actively with your healthcare provider, making informed choices about your lifestyle, and monitoring your body's responses are all integral steps that empower you to manage your bipolar disorder effectively while maintaining the highest possible quality of life. Make sure to keep yourself informed, asking your doctor questions for information on the drug as well as potential side effects.

THE ROLE OF HOLISTIC THERAPIES IN TREATMENT PLANS

In the realm of treating bipolar disorder, holistic therapies offer a complement to traditional medical treatments, providing a broader approach to wellness that addresses the symptoms and the overall well-being of individuals. These therapies, which include acupuncture, yoga, and meditation, have gained recognition for their effectiveness in reducing symptoms of mental health disorders and enhancing overall health and stress management. Let's explore how these therapies work, the evidence supporting their use, and how you can integrate them into your existing treatment plan.

Acupuncture involves the insertion of fine needles into specific points of the body. Clinical studies have shown that acupuncture can help alleviate the symptoms of depression and anxiety, common companions of bipolar disorder. Yoga, a practice that dates back thousands of years, has been shown to significantly impact mental health. Regular yoga practice has been associated with reductions in stress, better mood and emotional regulation, and an overall enriched quality of life (Madeson, 2024). Meditation, particularly mindfulness meditation, involves focusing your attention while keeping an open mind and eliminating environmental and mental distractions. Research supports the use of mindfulness in reducing the symptoms of anxiety and depression, improving emotional regulation, and increasing resilience to stress (Miller, 2019).

Research has shown that holistic therapies and their effectiveness in treating mental health symptoms have a promising future. It can reduce symptoms in a variety of ways, such as decreasing stress and helping to manage stress and anxiety. In fact, it can even help with chronic pain associated with mental health and trauma. The management of depression and anxiety, which are both symptoms of bipolar, can be especially effective. Students in a research study reported feeling more in control of their health, being able to handle stressful events, and taking responsibility for themselves and their well-being (Madeson, 2024).

Incorporating holistic therapies into your treatment strategy can provide a multi-faceted approach to managing bipolar disorder, one that nurtures both the body and the mind. As you consider these options, remember that the most effective treatment plan is one that is tailored to your unique needs and life circumstances, embracing a comprehensive approach to health and wellness. Integrating these holistic therapies into a treatment plan should be done thoughtfully and preferably under the guidance of your healthcare provider. It is important to view these therapies as complementary to, not replacements for, traditional medical treatments such as medication and psychotherapy (Mayo Clinic, 2024).

The personal stories of those who have integrated holistic therapies into their treatment plans often highlight profound benefits. Take, for example, a patient named Sarah, who found that yoga helped stabilize her moods. She utilized acupuncture alongside medication to manage her bipolar symptoms, noting a significant reduction in her mood events and a boost in her overall sense of well-being. As you can see, there are real-life, tangible stories of how holistic therapy, especially when integrated with traditional medicine, can positively impact your life (Clear Mind Treatment, 2024).

There are many ways to treat and manage bipolar disorder and its symptoms. Integrating holistic approaches alongside traditional medicine can increase overall quality of life. Research has discovered a positive future for these treatment modalities. Tailoring your plan for your specific needs, including both holistic and traditional medicine, under the guidance of your doctor, is a positive step in managing your bipolar.

WHEN TO CONSIDER HOSPITALIZATION: GUIDANCE AND PREPARATION

In managing bipolar disorder, most treatment occurs in outpatient settings, which allows you to maintain your regular lifestyle while receiving treatment. However, there are times when outpatient care might not be sufficient, particularly during severe episodes of mania or depression. Understanding when hospitalization is necessary, what it involves, and how to prepare for it can make this process less daunting and more effective in stabilizing your condition. It is important to keep an open mind, especially when it comes to the stigma around bipolar and hospitalization for mental health. Your health is paramount.

Hospitalization may become necessary when symptoms become severe enough to pose a danger to yourself or others or when you are unable to care for yourself. This can include instances of psychosis and problematic behaviors. During major depressive episodes, hospitalization might be required if there is a risk of self-harm or suicide or if you become too incapacitated by your depression to manage daily activities. If you present a danger to yourself and/or others, you may need hospitalization as well. The goal of hospitalization is to provide a safe environment where intensive treatment can stabilize your condition quickly. How long you stay is often determined by a mental health professional who will help establish a plan to support and keep you safe after discharge (Moore, 2022).

The experience of being hospitalized for bipolar disorder can vary, but it generally includes a combination of medication management, psychotherapy, and support in a controlled environment. Upon admission, a detailed assessment of your mental health will be conducted to tailor an immediate treatment plan. A medical evaluation will follow to determine if there are any underlying medical conditions that may be related to your symptoms. It is important to remember that hospital stays can stir up strong emotions as it may be tough to be outside of your environment. After evaluation, the mental health professionals you are working with will determine a treatment plan and how long you will stay (Moore, 2022).

Preparing for the possibility of hospitalization, though hoping it may never be necessary, is a practical step you can take. Preparing a 'hospital bag' with essentials such as clothes, personal hygiene items, and perhaps a comforting personal item like a book or a photo can ease the stress if hospitalization becomes necessary (Turner, 2023). In my experience, it is also wise to discuss plans with your employer and family to manage your responsibilities during your absence, guaranteeing your obligations are covered without added stress. It is important to develop an understanding of your insurance coverage for hospitalization as that can alleviate financial worries, providing you with clear information on what treatments are covered and any out-of-pocket costs you may expect.

Post-hospitalization care is crucial and involves a structured plan for transitioning back to community living. This plan usually includes follow-up appointments with your mental health provider, ongoing medication management, and recommendations for therapy. Adjustments to your treatment plan will likely be made based on your response to treatment during your stay. It is important that you have a thorough understanding of your discharge plan and are on board. Your participation is crucial to the success of the plan and to maintaining or improving your health (Magellan Healthcare, 2020).

Hospitalization for bipolar disorder can be a pivotal intervention in times of severe crisis. It provides an intensive level of care aimed at stabilizing severe symptoms quickly. While the prospect of hospitalization can be intimidating, understanding when it is necessary, what to expect, and how to prepare can help you approach it as a constructive part of your overall treatment plan. Remember, this level of care is about providing you the support you need to regain stability and continue your path toward long-term management of bipolar disorder. It will help you thrive and enhance your quality of life.

In this chapter, we have explored the array of treatment options available for managing bipolar disorder. Understanding your options, how they work together, and when each is appropriate allows you to handle your treatment with greater confidence. As we continue, the next chapter will discover the crucial roles that support systems and relationships play in managing bipolar disorder, highlighting how interconnected support networks are not just beneficial but essential for those living with this condition.

CHAPTER 4

SUPPORT SYSTEMS AND RELATIONSHIPS

When living with bipolar disorder, your support network acts as your lighthouse, providing guidance, safety, and reassurance through turbulent times. Building a robust support network is not merely about gathering people around you; it involves carefully choosing those who understand the complexities of bipolar disorder, are committed to your well-being, and can positively impact your path toward stability.

BUILDING A RELIABLE SUPPORT NETWORK

Creating a strong support network requires patience, care, and thoughtful consideration of who will best thrive in the environment you provide and who, in turn, will support your growth. Surrounding yourself with people who are open to educating themselves about the disorder is critical. However, it is important to set boundaries and communicate expectations to help avoid additional stress and maintain a sense of personal space. Engaging with your support network will help you maintain control over your bipolar disorder. In this section, we will explore these topics further, helping you develop a support network of your own.

The first step in cultivating this is identifying potential members who can contribute positively to your wellness. I have personally spent a significant amount of time building my support plan. This can include family and friends, mental health professionals, or established support groups. Each of these options brings a unique perspective and set of resources that can assist you in different aspects of your life. In fact, you might find a combination of those options to be most successful.

Educating your network is crucial. We understand that knowledge is power, but it is more than that. It is also empathy. Not everyone will understand what bipolar disorder entails, and misconceptions are common. Take the time to share resources, such as books and articles, or even direct them to educational workshops about bipolar disorder in order to cultivate a deep understanding of the disorder. This education can transform their support from well-meaning but ineffective to empowering and insightful (Etcheson, 2021).

Setting clear boundaries and expectations with your support network is essential for maintaining a healthy dynamic that respects your personal space and emotional needs. This might involve communicating your needs and expectations. While boundaries will vary according to the person and the situation, it often means communicating what is or is not acceptable for you. For example, if you have a loved one who often uses you as a sounding board every evening after work, but you need that time to cool down from the day. In this situation, you would need to communicate that you need to find a more convenient time to talk because, while you are happy to talk, you need quiet time in the evenings. This validates the needs and feelings of the other person, setting a boundary that fulfills your needs and wants as well. Setting boundaries is an important part of managing your bipolar disorder and relationships. Research has shown that maintaining your boundaries has numerous benefits, so it is important that these boundaries are communicated clearly and revisited often, as your needs may change over time (Cohen, 2024).

Regular engagement with your support network is vital. Make a habit of checking in with your support system regularly. This could be in the form of regular updates via phone calls, messages, or in-person meetings. Keeping your network informed of your status and goals helps in maintaining the connection and confirms they are prepared and proactive rather than reactive, which can significantly affect the effectiveness of their support (Mihajlovic, 2024). A support network is a crucial part of healing, allowing you to manage your disorder more effectively. Take care of who you select to be in your support system, as their participation will impact your well-being. Remember to communicate honestly and openly about your needs and expectations. With a support system in place, you will find a better quality of life is right around the corner.

COMMUNICATION STRATEGIES FOR DISCUSSING BIPOLAR DISORDER

As I mentioned in the previous section, communication is a key part of managing your bipolar alongside your support team. It is important to be mindful of the language you are using when communicating with others. The time and place you say things is also critical. For example, if you were upset by a friend who may have said something hurtful, you will want to talk to them.

However, doing it at a mutual friend's wedding is not the right time or place. Instead, you would meet privately and discuss the matter. Communication is most effective when practiced with an open mind and honest heart, especially when discussing difficult topics. Let's further discuss these points.

When it comes to discussing bipolar disorder, the words you choose and the way you communicate can profoundly impact the understanding and support you receive from others. Using respectful and non-stigmatizing language is paramount. Words have power—they can shape perceptions, influence emotions, and either build bridges or create barriers. When talking about bipolar disorder, it is vital to use terms that convey the medical nature of the condition, avoiding colloquialisms or derogatory terms that perpetuate stigma (Richards, 2018).

Choosing the right time and setting for these discussions is equally crucial. The goal is to make sure the conversation is both productive and comfortable. It is important to talk about your condition when you are stable; however, when your symptoms worsen, there are a few signs that it might be time to talk. For example, when your thoughts and feelings start to become abnormal and affect your day-to-day life. If your symptoms persist, it is important to communicate with your support system (Mental Health America, n.d.).

Since my diagnosis, I have learned how important healthy communication is. Being open and honest about your feelings and experiences with bipolar disorder can significantly deepen the understanding and connection between you and your listener. It is important to express the clinical aspects of the disorder, like how it impacts your daily life, your relationships, and your emotional well-being. Honesty inspires trust and empathy, which are crucial for building supportive relationships. However, it is also important to gauge how much to share and with whom; being selective about sharing personal details can protect your emotional health and verify your openness is respected and valued.

Handling difficult questions or reactions requires patience and preparedness. Not everyone will respond positively or understandingly; some may ask invasive questions or react in ways that feel dismissive or judgmental. Preparing for these possibilities can help you respond calmly and effectively. Try to listen to the person actively, which allows you to hear their side and respond appropriately (Mind, n.d.). I have found it is important to understand that everyone has a different experience with mental health and may need more support and education in order to process these difficult questions and topics.

Each of these strategies is a step toward more meaningful and supportive communications. By choosing your words carefully, setting the right scene, being open in a measured way, and handling tricky interactions with grace, you can better your relationships and create a supportive network that truly understands and respects your bipolar disorder diagnosis.

HOW PARTNERS CAN SUPPORT DURING MOOD EPISODES

Traversing the complexities of bipolar disorder requires self-awareness and the informed, compassionate involvement of those closest to you, particularly your partner. Understanding how to effectively support a loved one during mood episodes can significantly advance the relationship's strength and the well-being of both individuals involved.

A crucial aspect of this support is the ability to recognize the early signs of mood episodes. For a partner, this might mean noticing subtle changes in behavior, energy levels, or sleep patterns that precede a manic or depressive episode. These signs can vary widely; while one person may exhibit increased irritability or restlessness as they approach a manic episode, another might begin withdrawing socially as a precursor to depression (Mayo Clinic, n.d.). Partners can prepare by educating themselves, learning your warning signs, and discussing them openly to develop a mutual understanding of potential indicators. Partners can help implement an established episode plan, confirm any adjustments to your treatment plan are made, and support you in managing your symptoms (Martin, 2021).

Effective communication during these episodes plays a pivotal role. Techniques such as active listening, where the partner provides full attention, refrains from judgment, and responds in a way that acknowledges the emotions being expressed, can be particularly beneficial. It is also helpful to ask direct but gentle questions that encourage the person to express what they are feeling and what they need, rather than making assumptions, but they should avoid asking too many (Mind, n.d.).

In terms of practical help, there are several ways partners can be supportive during mood episodes. Providing general support, such as taking over certain responsibilities, especially those that might add stress or require a level of focus that the person may not currently possess, can be a huge relief. Establishing medication adherence is another critical area where partners can assist. This might involve reminding the person to take their medication or attending doctor's appointments with them to stay informed about their treatment plan. Such support helps in managing the disorder. It reinforces a nurturing relationship where both partners feel involved and valued (International Bipolar Foundation, n.d.).

Providing emotional support while maintaining respect for the individual's space and condition is perhaps one of the most delicate aspects of supporting a partner through a mood episode. This support might look different depending on the phase of the episode. It is crucial to maintain a balance between offering support and respecting the individual's need for space (International Bipolar Foundation, n.d.).

Supporting a partner with bipolar disorder during mood episodes is a nuanced dance that requires patience, understanding, and proactive communication. By learning to recognize the early signs of mood episodes, communicating effectively, providing practical help, and offering emotional support, partners can play a crucial role in managing the disorder. This collaborative approach helps in getting through the episodes more smoothly, strengthening the relationship and building a foundation of mutual support and understanding that extends beyond the challenges of bipolar disorder. With the support of your partner, you will find yourself well on your way to improving your quality of life.

NAVIGATING BIPOLAR DISORDER WITH CHILDREN IN THE FAMILY

As we have discussed, bipolar disorder most often manifests during early adulthood. However, it can affect people of all ages, including children. In this section, we will discuss how it impacts them and how to best support them. Through maintaining routines and modeling healthy behaviors, you can provide the care the child needs, helping them manage their disorder and live a full life.

Explaining bipolar disorder to children requires a delicate balance of simplicity and honesty, checking that the information is both comprehensible and age appropriate. Initiating a conversation about bipolar disorder with a child involves breaking down the complexities of the condition into terms they can grasp. Make sure you discuss the essentials, helping them understand the chronic condition. Keep your child's age in mind as you do this, and only provide as much information as they can understand. Allow your child to ask questions, helping them understand the situation to the best of their ability. For adolescents who can understand more nuanced explanations, you might describe how everyone's brain has chemicals that affect how they feel, and sometimes, these chemicals can become imbalanced, leading to the symptoms of bipolar disorder. Regardless of the child's age, reassure them that it is not anyone's fault, emphasizing that just like any illness, bipolar disorder requires understanding, care, and sometimes medication to manage (Jensen, 2023).

In earlier chapters, we discussed the importance of routine for those with bipolar disorder. Routines create a sense of predictability and security, which can be particularly comforting to children in an environment that may sometimes feel chaotic. This includes consistent bedtime rituals and a structured schedule for homework and leisure activities. In my experience, even when bipolar disorder induces disruptions in the family's dynamics, striving to keep these routines intact can offer children a reliable framework that supports their daily lives. It may also be beneficial to involve children in the creation of these routines, which can expand their sense of control and inclusion, making the routines more meaningful and easier to adhere to (Currin-Sheehan, 2021).

Support for children in families dealing with bipolar disorder is crucial and can take many forms, from emotional support within the family to professional counseling. Encouraging open communication within the family allows children to express their feelings and concerns about the bipolar disorder affecting their loved ones. Professional counseling can also be invaluable, providing children with a safe space to discuss their feelings with an impartial adult. This can be particularly helpful when children need to cope with complex emotions they might not yet fully understand or feel comfortable discussing at home. Support groups designed for families dealing with mental health issues can also offer a communal sense of understanding and acceptance, showing children that they are not alone and that other families face similar challenges (Grey, 2023).

Role modeling effective coping skills is a powerful teaching tool for children. Demonstrating techniques such as mindfulness, positive self-talk, and other healthy coping skills can equip children with tools to manage their own mental health from a young age. Furthermore, showing children that it is possible to live a fulfilling life despite the challenges of bipolar disorder instills hope and a positive outlook on managing personal adversities they may encounter in the future (Klein-Baer, n.d.).

Finding your way through bipolar disorder in a family setting, especially with children, involves an ongoing commitment to communication, education, and support. By taking proactive steps, you can develop an environment that supports the well-being of the child. It strengthens the family unit, making it better equipped to handle the complexities of bipolar disorder. This approach helps in managing the immediate impacts of the disorder and lays down a foundation of understanding and resilience that children can carry into their own futures.

WORKPLACE DYNAMICS: ADVOCATING FOR YOURSELF PROFESSIONALLY

Plotting a course through the professional world while managing bipolar disorder can be difficult. It involves making informed decisions about disclosure, understanding your legal rights, developing supportive relationships with HR, and maintaining a balance that prevents work-related triggers. These elements are crucial for creating a work environment where you can thrive without fear of stigma or misunderstanding.

The decision to disclose your bipolar disorder at work is highly personal and can have significant implications. There are a number of factors that may impact your decision. For example, women are less likely to disclose their condition than others. If you work in a supportive workplace and have a good relationship with your supervisor and coworkers, you might feel more comfortable. Perhaps your symptoms are affecting your work life, and you need accommodations to maintain your efficiency and productivity. This might be a challenge if you are strongly concerned with your professional status. Whatever the factors may be, it is important to weigh them and decide what's best for your specific situation (Seven, 2023).

Understanding and leveraging your legal protections under employment law is crucial. In many places, laws such as the Americans with Disabilities Act (ADA) in the United States provide protection against discrimination for individuals with disabilities, including those with mental illnesses like bipolar disorder. These laws also require employers to provide reasonable accommodations. These accommodations are designed to enable you to perform your job effectively without exacerbating your condition. Familiarize yourself with the specific provisions of these laws and consider seeking advice from legal experts or advocacy groups if you need guidance on how to assert your rights (U.S. Equal Employment Opportunity Commission, n.d.).

Building a positive and supportive relationship with your Human Resources (HR) department can significantly facilitate the process of negotiating accommodations. HR professionals are typically trained to handle sensitive personal information confidentially and to help implement workplace accommodations. Approach your HR representative with a clear outline of what accommodations you believe will assist you in performing your job effectively. Be prepared to explain how these accommodations will support your health and the productivity and quality of your work. It is helpful to have medical documentation that supports your request, as this can provide HR with the necessary information to understand and process your accommodations. Keeping open communication with your HR department can help make sure your needs are met.

Managing workload and stress is another critical aspect of thriving professionally. Work-related stress can be a significant trigger for mood episodes, so it is important to develop strategies to manage your workload effectively. Create boundaries between your work and personal lives and avoid doing work-related tasks after the workday has ended. Learn to recognize when you are overextended and be proactive in seeking adjustments or support. Regular breaks, even short ones, can significantly reduce stress levels and optimize overall productivity (Cherry, 2023).

Finding a way to explore the complexities of the workplace while managing bipolar disorder can help create a better quality of life. By making informed decisions about disclosure, utilizing your legal rights, engaging with HR, and managing your workload, you can create a professional environment that supports rather than hinders your health and productivity. This proactive approach benefits your career, contributing to your overall stability and wellness.

FINDING AND UTILIZING SUPPORT GROUPS AND ONLINE RESOURCES

For many steering through the complex emotions and challenges of bipolar disorder, support groups represent a vital component of their overall management strategy. These groups provide a unique environment where you can connect with others who truly understand the ups and downs of living with bipolar disorder. It is important to find the right group, whether it is online or in-person, and keep safety and privacy in mind. From there, you should be able to find a support group that fits your needs. Let's learn more about finding the right fit and how that will benefit you.

The benefits of such groups are manifold. Sharing your experiences with others who have similar stories can validate your feelings, which is often a profound relief. You can grow through the experiences you share with the group. Furthermore, these groups can be a wellspring of practical advice, helping you to learn better coping strategies and practice better self-care. The emotional support offered in these settings can be particularly powerful, providing both comfort and hope during tough periods (Hoy, n.d.).

Choosing the right support group is crucial and should be approached with thoughtful consideration. The focus of the group should align with your needs. There are a variety of group types, such as mutual support groups and therapy groups. The format of the group also matters—whether it is in-person or online. In-person groups offer a sense of immediacy and personal connection, while online groups provide flexibility and accessibility, particularly if you live in an area where in-person groups are limited or if your schedule makes attending regular meetings challenging (Hoy, n.d.). Additionally, I have found it is important to consider the background of the facilitator; an experienced leader, possibly with professional training in mental health, can guarantee discussions remain helpful and that the group provides a safe and supportive environment.

Utilizing online resources effectively can also significantly heighten your ability to manage bipolar disorder. The internet is a treasure trove of information, offering access to a wide range of forums, educational websites, and social media groups dedicated to bipolar disorder. Websites run by reputable health organizations, such as the International Bipolar Foundation, can provide up-to-date medical information and treatment options, helping you stay informed about the latest research and therapies. Online forums and social media groups offer opportunities to ask questions, share experiences, and receive support at any time of day, which can be incredibly helpful during times when you are seeking immediate advice or feeling isolated.

However, traversing online spaces requires careful consideration of safety and privacy. When participating in forums and social media, it is important to protect your personal information. Avoid sharing identifiable details such as your full name, address, birth date, or specific details of your workplace. Always check the privacy settings of the online platforms you use to understand who can see your posts and comments. It is best to assume there is not privacy and act accordingly (Forbes Technology Council, 2019).

Engaging with support groups and utilizing online resources can provide you with a network of support and a wealth of information, making a significant difference in how you manage bipolar disorder. Finding others in similar situations dealing with the same disorder can help you feel less alone, and you can manage it better when you are educated about the disorder and treatment options. These resources empower you not just to survive but to thrive, offering support that is both accessible and aligned with your needs.

In this chapter, we explored the invaluable role of support systems and relationships in managing bipolar disorder. From building a reliable support network to effectively communicating about your condition, each aspect plays a crucial role in enhancing your stability and quality of life. As we transition to the next chapter, we will begin looking into coping mechanisms and resilience building, essential skills that will further empower you to face the complexities of bipolar disorder with confidence and hope.

RAISING AWARENESS

"What mental health needs is more sunlight, more candor, and more unashamed conversation."

— GLENN CLOSE

There's a much greater awareness and understanding of mental health than there has been in the past, yet no matter how much more accepting the world becomes, living with bipolar disorder will always be a little scary. Whether you live it with yourself or you're caring for someone who does, the chances are, you've had experiences that have unsettled you. Understanding the condition is the key to removing this fear—and that's when we can make real progress.

I was diagnosed with bipolar disorder five years ago, and that diagnosis brought a mixed bag of feelings, but one of them was relief. Understanding that there was a name for what was happening to me and being able to make sense of the experiences that had terrified me in the past was a huge blessing, and it empowered me to learn more about the condition and how it affected me—and that brought with it so many rewards that I'm determined to share what I've learned with others. This is how it is that you come to be reading this book, and I hope that through it, you'll be able to access the same opportunities for growth that I have.

In 2019, 40 million people were living with bipolar disorder (World Health Organization, 2022): There are clearly many people who would benefit from deepening their understanding and learning more about what they can do to navigate its challenges. I want to reach as many of those people as I can, and you can help me.

By leaving a review of this book on Amazon, you'll help it reach the people who are looking for it, bringing peace of mind and an improved quality of life to more people.

It's through reviews that books find their way into the hands of the people they're meant for, so a few words from you could make a huge difference.

There's no shame in living with any kind of mental health disorder; let's try to raise awareness and help more people to navigate it with confidence. Thank you so much for your support.

Scan the QR code below:

CHAPTER 5
COPING MECHANISMS AND RESILIENCE BUILDING

Individuals with bipolar disorder have the unique opportunity to transform challenges into triumphs through effective coping mechanisms and resilience building. This chapter is dedicated to empowering you with cognitive strategies and practical tools that will guide you in sculpting a resilient and fulfilling life despite the ebbs and flows of bipolar disorder.

COGNITIVE BEHAVIORAL TECHNIQUES FOR MOOD MANAGEMENT

As you have learned, Cognitive Behavioral Therapy (CBT) is particularly effective for managing bipolar disorder, as it addresses the negative thinking patterns that can lead to or exacerbate mood swings. In this section, we will dive into the techniques you can learn to help you regulate your emotions and reduce mood episodes (American Psychological Association, n.d.). From mindfulness to incorporating the techniques into your day-to-day management routine, there are plenty of ways to benefit from CBT.

CBT offers a toolbox of techniques that you can use to modify problematic thoughts and behaviors. There are some physical practices you can try. For example, mindful breathing can help keep you calm and focused. Trying progressive muscle relaxation can help you reduce tension in your body and provide a sense of calmness. CBT will help you address and deconstruct cognitive distortions. Cognitive restructuring, one of these techniques, involves identifying and challenging the irrational or harmful thoughts that often arise during mood episodes. You might even take up journaling, which can help identify patterns of thoughts and behaviors (Ackerman, 2017).

Consider the example of Maria, who often found herself immobilized by depression and negative thoughts about her self-worth. Through CBT, Maria learned to recognize and challenge these harmful thoughts. She replaced them with affirmations of her strengths and achievements, which she wrote down and reviewed daily, giving her the additional benefits offered by journaling. Additionally, Maria and her therapist identified activities that had historically made her feel good, such as painting and yoga. By planning and committing to these activities, even when her mood was low, Maria began to experience more frequent and longer-lasting periods of stability.

Integrating CBT with medication can significantly impact treatment outcomes for bipolar disorder. Medications tend to show results faster than CBT; however, research has shown that patients in CBT are less likely to experience returning symptoms if treatment is stopped. This combination allows for a more comprehensive approach to treatment: medication addresses the biological aspects of the disorder, while CBT helps modify the psychological patterns that contribute to mood instability (Association for Behavioral and Cognitive Therapies, n.d.).

Through the diligent application of CBT strategies, you can gain greater control over your thoughts and behaviors. This empowered approach to managing bipolar disorder reduces symptoms, building a foundation of skills that can support long-term wellness and resilience. As you continue to apply these strategies, remember that each step forward, no matter how small, is significant progress toward stability and wellness. In the next section, we will discuss how mindfulness and meditation can supplement these methods, bettering your overall experience.

MINDFULNESS AND MEDITATION: PRACTICES FOR FOCUS AND CALM

In the ebb and flow of emotions that characterize bipolar disorder, mindfulness acts as an anchor, offering a way to cultivate peace amid the chaos. This practice, which often includes meditation, is ancient. Mindfulness and meditation help center you and provide a sense of calm, making handling mood episodes easier. In this section, we will look at the benefits of these practices and how you can incorporate them into your routine.

Mindfulness is the practice of being fully present in the moment, aware of where you are and what you are doing, without becoming overly reactive or overwhelmed by what is going on around you. This practice holds profound benefits for individuals with bipolar disorder, particularly in its capacity to diminish stress and anxiety, improve emotional regulation, and increase overall mental health. It can even reduce symptoms of depression. By training the mind to focus on the present, mindfulness can help break the cycle of mood swings by providing a tool to manage reactions to emotional triggers (Cherry, 2022).

The essence of mindfulness lies in its simplicity and accessibility. It can be practiced through various forms, but some of the most effective are focused breathing exercises and body scans. Focused breathing involves concentrating on the breath, noticing the air entering and exiting the body, and using this focus to anchor the mind in the present moment. This practice can be particularly helpful when feelings of anxiety or mania begin to surface, acting as a natural relaxant (Riopel, 2019). A body scan is another mindfulness technique where you mentally scan yourself from head to toe, observing any discomfort, tension, or sensations you feel. This practice clarifies one's awareness of bodily sensations and a sense of physical and mental alignment (O'Bryan, 2021).

Mindfulness proves especially valuable during mood swings, which are a hallmark of bipolar disorder. During these times, mindfulness exercises can serve as a stabilizing force, helping you observe your emotions and thoughts without judgment. Mindfulness encourages a pause and a reflective moment where choices can be made about how to respond to big, unregulated feelings. This can lead to a more deliberate and less reactive approach to mood swings, potentially reducing their intensity and frequency. For instance, when you notice the onset of irritability or euphoria that might signal the beginning of a manic episode, taking time to engage in a mindfulness exercise can help modulate these emotions, keeping your mood more balanced. You can incorporate these practices into your everyday routine, mastering the skills so when mood swings occur, you are well-practiced and can respond appropriately (Hamilton, n.d.).

To further explore and deepen your mindfulness practice, numerous resources are available that cater to different preferences and needs. Apps like Headspace or Calm offer guided meditations, daily mindfulness exercises, and more, making it easy to integrate mindfulness into your daily routine (Blackwell, 2023). For those who prefer a more structured approach, there are many books on the practice of mindfulness and meditation. Books such as *Wherever You Go, There You Are* by Jon Kabat-Zinn can provide insights and practices to expand your understanding of mindfulness (Lamoreux, 2021). Additionally, local or online courses in mindfulness meditation can offer structured learning and support from experienced instructors, helping you cultivate a practice that can withstand the complexities of bipolar disorder. Online sites such as Coursera and Mindful offer courses that can help you learn more about the practices.

Incorporating mindfulness and meditation into your life offers a robust tool for managing bipolar disorder. It equips you with the means to remain centered and calm, regardless of external circumstances or internal emotions. Mood swings become more manageable as you develop healthy coping skills. As you continue to practice and integrate these techniques into your daily life, they can become invaluable tools as you work toward stability and peace.

THE ROLE OF JOURNALING IN EMOTIONAL CLARITY

With bipolar disorder, you often experience a lot of emotions, which can be hard to identify and process. When managing bipolar disorder, you might come across journaling as a coping tool. There are different types of journaling, which we will discuss later in this section. This variety allows you to find the journaling style that fits you best. With effective journaling, you can safely explore your emotions.

The act of journaling in the context of bipolar disorder involves cultivating a space where thoughts and feelings can be expressed and examined. This leads to greater understanding and management of the condition. Maintaining a daily journal allows you to track your mood patterns, identify triggers, and monitor your progress over time. This practice can be incredibly therapeutic, providing a private venue for externalizing thoughts and emotions that might be too complex or confusing to articulate verbally (Bedosky, 2024).

Journaling can serve various therapeutic purposes depending on the method employed. Gratitude journaling, for example, focuses on recording things you are thankful for each day (Bedosky, 2024). Symptom journaling involves documenting your daily symptoms. This type of journaling is invaluable for communicating effectively with your medical team, providing both you and your healthcare providers with detailed insights that can inform treatment adjustments (Crider, 2023). Free writing allows for unstructured expression of thoughts and feelings (Wagner, 2017).

There are some tricks to maximizing the therapeutic benefits of journaling. Writing regularly, ideally at the same time each day, helps in developing a routine that reinforces the habit of journaling (Bedosky, 2024). Being honest and reflective in your entries is equally important; the more truthful and introspective you are in your journal, the more useful it will be as a tool for self-discovery and management (Notebooks and Planners, 2023). Regularly reviewing past entries is another beneficial practice. This review can reveal progress that might not be evident day-to-day, reinforcing positive behaviors and highlighting areas that need adjustment (Faulkner, 2023).

The personal nature of a journal, particularly one that includes detailed accounts of your mental health, necessitates careful consideration of privacy and security. The thought of someone else reading your journal can be unsettling and may inhibit the honesty of your entries. Here are a few tips I have found helpful when trying to keep your journals safe and private. You might choose to keep your journal in a locked drawer or a safe. If you prefer digital journaling, numerous apps offer encryption and password protection to secure your entries. It is important to choose a reputable app that prioritizes user privacy and data security, verifying that your sensitive information is well protected.

Journaling plays a crucial role in managing bipolar disorder because it allows you to process and better understand thoughts and emotions. Regardless of what type of journaling you use, this practice offers a versatile and accessible means to heighten your emotional clarity and stability. By integrating journaling into your daily routine and adhering to practices that foster its effectiveness and security, you can harness this powerful tool to explore the complexities of bipolar disorder.

DEVELOPING PERSONAL CRISIS MANAGEMENT PLANS

Mental health conditions such as bipolar disorder often require crisis management plans. As you may have guessed, these plans help guarantee your health and safety in times of crisis. It is important to develop a plan that contains core components like warning signs and important phone numbers. It might take more than one attempt to get the plan right, but once you do, you can rest assured that you are prepared to manage your disorder even in times of high stress. Let's take a deeper look at how crisis management plans work.

Much like a safety drill, a personal crisis plan prepares you and your caregivers for the possibility of severe mood episodes, making sure everyone knows the steps to take to manage the situation effectively and safely. This proactive approach provides a structured response that can mitigate the intensity of the episode and potentially prevent hospitalization (Myers, 2020).

A robust crisis management plan is comprehensive and tailored to your specific needs and symptoms. It starts with the identification of warning signs and triggers that herald the onset of a severe manic or depressive episode. Next, the plan should outline clear, concrete steps to manage symptoms. This might include what helps calm you down and safety measures. For instance, you may have a designated "quiet room" in your home where you can go to feel safe and reduce sensory overload during manic episodes. Including essential contact information in your crisis plan is crucial. This list should include your psychiatrist, therapist, a trusted family member or friend, and a local emergency contact (Myers, 2020).

Caregivers play an invaluable role in your crisis management plan, acting as both observers and active participants in managing the situation. Their responsibilities can range from providing assistance with daily activities to executing specific parts of the plan, such as administering medication or contacting medical professionals. Caregivers can also provide emotional support (Schulz et al., 2016). It is important for caregivers to be well-informed about the specifics of the plan and comfortable with the responsibilities assigned to them. Regular discussions and walk-throughs of the plan can help verify everyone is prepared and confident in their roles, which can significantly smooth the process when a real crisis occurs.

Regularly reviewing and updating your crisis management plan is crucial to its effectiveness. As you progress in your treatment or as new insights are gained about your condition, adjustments might be necessary. Regular reviews—perhaps every six months or after a significant mood episode—make sure the plan adapts to your needs and remains a relevant and powerful tool in your management strategy. These updates should be done in consultation with your healthcare providers and caregivers to verify all perspectives are considered and that the plan adheres to the latest medical advice.

Creating and maintaining a personal crisis management plan empowers you to take control of your bipolar disorder, particularly during times when you might feel most vulnerable. This plan acts as a blueprint for you and your support network. It provides clear directives that can reduce the severity of mood episodes and protect your overall well-being. As you integrate this plan into your overall management strategy, let it serve as a testament to your commitment to living a balanced and healthy life. You can rest easy knowing you are equipped to handle the challenges that come with bipolar disorder.

OVERCOMING NEGATIVE THOUGHT PATTERNS

Negative thoughts can have a major impact on how you live your life. It is important to be able to recognize them when they appear and challenge them appropriately. This provides the space for you to practice more positive self-talk, which is especially effective when practiced regularly. Let's see how you can practice these skills and overcome negative thoughts.

The ability to identify and reshape negative thought patterns is akin to learning how to steer your way through a storm. Negative thoughts can contribute to feelings of worthlessness and anxiety, making it challenging to maintain emotional stability. Common cognitive distortions include rumination, where you fixate on negative thoughts, and catastrophizing, where you anticipate the worst possible outcome in a situation (Sutton, 2024).

Once you have identified these negative thoughts, the next step is to challenge and reframe them into more balanced and constructive ones. This process involves questioning the validity of your negative thoughts and replacing them with more realistic, balanced perspectives. You might start by simply noting down your thoughts whenever you feel a shift in your mood. Challenge your thoughts by checking the facts to see what the reality of the situation is. You can even use positive imagery and self-talk to shift the direction your thoughts are going in. Regardless of the technique, identifying and challenging thoughts can help (Sutton, 2024)

Building positive self-talk is another essential element in this process. Positive self-talk involves speaking to yourself in an optimistic manner, much as you would to a good friend. This might involve affirmations, which are positive statements that you repeat to yourself to encourage self-esteem and challenge negative patterns. Over time, these positive affirmations can become ingrained, gradually replacing the negative thought patterns that can trigger or worsen mood swings. As they become second nature, you will find your sense of confidence and resilience growing (Nash, 2019).

The transformation of thought patterns is not an overnight process but a continuous practice that requires patience and persistence. One effective way to cultivate this change is through regular mental exercises designed to build cognitive flexibility. For example, something as simple as meeting someone new can create an improvement in your brain. Setting aside a dedicated time each day for these practices can help integrate them into your routine, making them a regular part of your approach to managing bipolar disorder (Verdolin, 2019).

Engaging in these practices helps you challenge the negative thoughts you have and manage how they impact you more effectively. As you continue to apply these strategies and witness their benefits, you reinforce your commitment to nurturing a healthier mind, paving the way for long-term stability and resilience.

CELEBRATING SMALL WINS: BUILDING BLOCKS OF RESILIENCE

It can be difficult to manage the symptoms of bipolar disorder. When you struggle to manage your mood, it can be disappointing to feel like progress is slow. Instead of fixating on the negative, it is important to focus on the positives and the wins you achieve, both big and small.

Embracing each small achievement builds your confidence. It reinforces your motivation, creating a positive feedback loop that sustains your long-term management efforts. Setting achievable goals is the cornerstone of this approach. These goals should be specific, measurable, achievable, realistic, and time-bound (SMART) and tailored to align with your capabilities and current circumstances. We will discuss SMART goals later on. The key is to define these goals clearly, making them manageable enough to accomplish without overwhelming yourself. By setting achievable goals, you set yourself up for success (Mind Tools, n.d.).

Acknowledging and celebrating progress, no matter how modest, plays a crucial role in maintaining your morale and adherence to your management plan. It is essential to recognize that every step forward is a victory. Celebrating these achievements can be as simple as taking some time to reflect, sharing your progress with a friend or support group, or treating yourself to a favorite activity. Each celebration acts as a reinforcement, a reminder of your capabilities and progress, which can be particularly uplifting during times when you feel stuck or discouraged (Clarke, 2021).

Setbacks are an inevitable part of life, and more so when managing a condition like bipolar disorder. However, viewing setbacks not as failures but as opportunities for learning and growth can transform these experiences into valuable lessons. When a setback occurs, such as a missed goal or a challenging mood episode, it is helpful to approach it with curiosity rather than judgment. Analyze what might have contributed to the setback and identify areas for growth and development. It can be difficult to embrace failure and setbacks; however, it is a crucial part of growing. Remember, each setback is a stepping stone toward greater understanding and mastery of your condition (Bradley, 2023).

Sustaining momentum in your mental health management is crucial and can be achieved through continuous connection with your support networks and ongoing therapy. Staying connected with friends, family, or support groups provides you with a safe place to discuss your experiences with someone who cares about you. Continued therapy, whether through regular sessions with a mental health professional or participation in group therapy, offers professional guidance and insights that reinforce your coping strategies (World Health Organization, 2021). Moreover, I have found it important to be open to adjusting your management strategies based on your evolving needs or in response to new insights gained from therapy or personal reflection. This adaptive approach safeguards your strategies and their ability to remain effective and responsive to your current state, promoting long-term resilience and stability.

Embracing the practice of setting goals, celebrating small wins, learning from setbacks, and sustaining momentum builds a resilient framework for managing bipolar disorder. These practices empower you to take active control of your condition, promoting a sense of accomplishment and progress. Keeping a positive mentality on your path to managing bipolar is critical, and using these tools can help you along the way.

As we conclude this chapter, we reflect on the importance of celebrating small wins and learning from every experience. These practices are fundamental building blocks of a resilient life. By acknowledging each success, learning from every setback, and maintaining momentum, you strengthen your ability to handle the complexities of bipolar disorder with confidence and grace. Looking ahead, the next chapter will explore special considerations in bipolar disorder, delving into how various life stages and circumstances can impact management strategies, further enriching your toolkit for living well with bipolar disorder.

CHAPTER 6

SPECIAL CONSIDERATIONS IN BIPOLAR DISORDER

Living with bipolar disorder requires an awareness of the unique challenges that can arise under different circumstances. In this chapter, we will discuss the special considerations that are crucial for managing bipolar disorder, beginning by focusing on aspects that affect women, including hormonal changes and their implications throughout various life stages.

BIPOLAR DISORDER IN WOMEN: PREGNANCY AND HORMONAL EFFECTS

The sex you were assigned at birth can play a role in how your bipolar disorder manifests. With the possibility of pregnancy and the role hormones play, females and women often experience the disorder differently. It can be challenging to manage bipolar through pregnancy, especially with postpartum factors to consider. How these factors are managed in the long run affects a woman's ability to manage her bipolar disorder. As we continue, we will take a more in-depth look at these factors at play.

The dance of hormones in a woman's body plays a crucial role not just in reproductive health but also in mood regulation. For women with bipolar disorder, understanding and managing these hormonal fluctuations is key to maintaining stability. Hormonal changes during menstrual cycles, pregnancy, and menopause can significantly impact mood stability. These fluctuations are primarily due to changes in estrogen and progesterone, hormones that have been shown to affect neurotransmitter systems involved in mood disorders (Wisner, 2023).

Dealing with pregnancy while managing bipolar disorder presents a unique set of challenges and considerations. The decision to maintain or adjust medication during pregnancy is critical and should be made with careful consideration of the potential risks and benefits. Many medications used in the treatment of bipolar disorder, including certain mood stabilizers like lithium and Depakote, can have dangerous implications for fetal health. However, discontinuing medication increases the risk of relapse during pregnancy and postpartum periods when women are particularly vulnerable to mood episodes. It is imperative to consult with healthcare providers to tailor a treatment plan that protects the safety and well-being of both mother and child. This may include monitoring and adjusting medications, increasing the frequency of psychotherapy sessions, and implementing additional support systems (Cherney, 2017).

Postpartum periods require special attention as women with bipolar disorder are at a higher risk for postpartum psychosis and depression. Preventive measures can be highly effective and include proactive management plans established during pregnancy. These plans involve the continuation or adjustment of medication under medical supervision, addressing safety concerns, and establishing robust support systems to help the new mother manage sleep deprivation and stress, both of which can significantly impact mood stability (Pedersen, 2022).

Long-term hormonal management is another vital aspect of care for women with bipolar disorder. Hormone therapy, a treatment where medications are used to regulate your body's hormone levels, can have interactions with medications used for bipolar disorder. It is essential to approach hormone therapy with caution. A holistic approach that includes regular assessments of hormone levels, psychiatric symptoms, and medication interactions, guided by both a gynecologist and a psychiatrist, can help in effectively managing these complex interactions (NeuroLaunch, 2023).

As we explore these nuanced aspects of bipolar disorder, it is clear that the path requires careful navigation. For women, understanding the interplay between hormonal changes and mood stability is crucial. By addressing these specific needs with tailored strategies and informed healthcare decisions, you can manage your condition effectively, making sure each step you take is grounded in knowledge and proactive care.

THE IMPACT OF AGING ON BIPOLAR DISORDER

As time passes, the nature of bipolar disorder develops, subtly shifting its expression and challenges. Aging brings wisdom and complexity, especially for those managing bipolar disorder. There are many factors involved in managing bipolar disorder as you age. You will experience different symptoms and challenges that might require adjustments to your treatment plan and support system. Aging is inevitable, so it is important that you prepare appropriately to continue living your best life.

One notable shift is in the symptom profile. Typically, the fiery mania of youth might give way to more depressive episodes as one grows older. These depressive periods tend to be longer and can merge subtly with the normal concerns of aging, such as worries about health and independence, making them harder to distinguish and treat. It is also been shown that mood episodes may increase as you age; however, you are less likely to become suicidal compared to younger people suffering from the disorder (Gurarie, 2024).

The challenges for older adults living with bipolar disorder are complex. One significant concern is the increased susceptibility to side effects from medications. In more advanced stages of life, your metabolism will change, which adds to the issue of raised side effects. Moreover, the presence of comorbidities complicates things further. It is not uncommon for an older adult to manage bipolar disorder and other chronic conditions like anxiety. Each condition might require medications that can interact unpredictably, complicating the management of bipolar disorder (Gurarie, 2024).

Adjusting treatment strategies for older adults requires a nuanced approach that considers these complexities. This adjustment is not merely about changing prescriptions but involves a holistic view of the individual's health. Polypharmacy, the use of multiple medications for treating various ailments, becomes a critical concern. Each added medication increases the risk of adverse interactions (Kurczewska-Michalak et al., 2021). Besides pharmacological adjustments, there is a need to monitor cognitive decline closely. Regular cognitive assessments can help in tailoring interventions that address both cognitive and mood stability. While there are no standardized treatments for cognitive decline, research shows that treatments for bipolar have varying records of effectiveness, still allowing for some prevention (Gurarie, 2024).

Support systems for aging individuals with bipolar disorder need particular attention. As physical health may decline and mobility becomes limited, the role of caregivers and support networks becomes increasingly critical. Building and maintaining these support systems involves establishing that caregivers are informed and educated about the nuances of bipolar disorder in the context of aging. Verifying boundaries are present and respected is crucial as it allows the individual with bipolar disorder to make decisions on their own. These systems offer practical assistance during times of need (Muinos, 2023).

Exploring the golden years with bipolar disorder calls for an adaptive approach that respects the changing dynamics of aging. By acknowledging these shifts and planning for them proactively, you can maintain a quality of life that honors both your experience and your wisdom. Keep an open mind toward adjusting your management plan as necessary and try to get ahead of it. This proactive stance provides hope that aging is not just about looking back but also moving forward with grace and stability.

SUBSTANCE USE AND BIPOLAR DISORDER: NAVIGATING DUAL DIAGNOSIS

When you or someone you love lives with bipolar disorder, encountering substance use as a co-occurring issue is not uncommon. It is important to handle these situations with care and empathy, understanding addiction as a disease and educating yourself just as you would about bipolar disorder. While challenges are present, there are strategies and prevention plans to help overcome them. Taking a dive into these topics will help you prepare to manage both bipolar disorder and substance abuse.

A dual diagnosis of substance abuse and bipolar disorder may be less prevalent than initially anticipated. Patients with both diagnoses can often have the symptoms of bipolar disorder manifest earlier than those without the comorbidity. The poor health outcomes associated with substance abuse disorders are a larger concern than the potential for mood events. However, mental health conditions can exasperate substance abuse issues. For example, individuals with comorbidity may increase abuse when coming out of a depressed episode (Ostacher, 2011).

The relationship between bipolar disorder and substance use is often bidirectional. As we just discussed, the mood swings associated with bipolar disorder can make the escape offered by substances seem appealing as a temporary relief from emotional turmoil. Traditional treatment methods that address only one condition often fall short, leaving the other to fester and undermine overall recovery efforts. Research shows that it is important to treat bipolar, regardless of the substance abuse comorbidity. This dual diagnosis can profoundly impact treatment outcomes, adding layers of complexity to both the management of bipolar disorder and recovery from addiction (Ostacher, 2011).

Managing cravings and avoiding triggers is another vital aspect of treatment for dual diagnosis. Behavioral therapies have proven effective in helping individuals understand and change the behaviors and thought patterns that lead to substance use. These therapies also equip you with strategies to cope with the cravings and emotional distress that can trigger substance use. Support groups can also offer a community of peers who understand the unique challenges of maneuvering through both bipolar disorder and substance use, providing a network of support and accountability. It is also important to lean on your support system and keep them informed of your situation, allowing them to help you manage your triggers and ride out the urge to relapse or act out (Wright, 2021).

Recovery from a dual diagnosis of bipolar disorder and substance use requires a comprehensive and sustained approach. Relapse prevention is a critical component, involving regular monitoring and adjustments to the treatment plan as needed. This ongoing process includes continuing therapy to learn skills and cope. Lifestyle modifications also play a significant role in recovery. See the section on the importance of routine in Chapter Two. Additionally, you should emphasize the practice of self-care and honesty, which are essential for long-term recovery (Melemis, 2015).

Traversing the path of dual diagnosis is undoubtedly complex, but with the right strategies and support, recovery and stability are achievable. With the assistance of your medical team and support system, you can build a foundation for a healthier and more stable life. As you continue to explore and apply these strategies, remember that each step forward is a move toward greater understanding and control over your health and life.

SEASONAL AFFECTIVE DISORDER AND BIPOLAR: MANAGING SEASONAL CHANGES

As the seasons shift, bringing about changes in daylight and weather patterns, many individuals experience shifts in their mood and energy levels. For those with bipolar disorder, these seasonal changes can be particularly challenging, as they may exacerbate symptoms or trigger new episodes. It is important to understand how these disorders interact with one another and how to manage them.

Seasonal Affective Disorder (SAD) is a type of depression that occurs at the same time each year and can significantly complicate the management of bipolar disorder. The reduction in sunlight during winter can lead to a drop in serotonin levels and disrupt the body's internal clock, which can lead to feelings of depression. For individuals with bipolar disorder, these changes can intensify depressive episodes or, conversely, may lead to manic episodes as seasons change toward spring and increased daylight (Cox, 2023).

Addressing the challenges posed by SAD involves a multi-layered approach. Light therapy, also known as phototherapy, has been shown to be an effective treatment for SAD. Light therapy involves exposure to a bright light that mimics natural sunlight, typically from a light box, which can influence brain chemicals linked to mood. The therapy usually starts with a daily session of about 30 minutes, ideally in the morning, to help regulate the body's circadian rhythms and boost serotonin levels. While light therapy is generally safe and has minimal side effects, potential side effects include eyestrain, headache, irritability, or nausea, all of which should be monitored (Vanbuskirk, 2023). It is a great way to get the benefits of the sun when time outside is scarce.

In addition to light therapy, making specific lifestyle adjustments can significantly mitigate the effects of seasonal changes. Seeking sunlight is an excellent way to brighten your mood. This can involve arranging your living and workspaces to receive maximum natural light during the day or using a light therapy box. Regular physical exercise, such as yoga, is also beneficial. Engaging in outdoor activities during daylight hours. Maintaining social activities is equally important. Planning regular social interactions, whether in person or virtually, can provide support and reduce feelings of loneliness and isolation (DiPirro, 2020).

The changing seasons can also necessitate adjustments in medication. For some, changes in mood patterns related to seasonal shifts may require modifications in the dosage or type of medication used. This should always be done under the careful supervision of a healthcare provider. It is crucial to remember that it can take weeks to see the full effects of the medication, so communicate openly with your doctor about any significant shifts you notice. Your healthcare provider might adjust your treatment plan accordingly, perhaps prescribing an antidepressant during the seasons you are affected by. This proactive approach can help prevent the onset of severe episodes and maintain stability throughout the year (Mayo Clinic, n.d.).

Dealing with the complexities of bipolar disorder with the added variable of seasonal changes demands an adaptive and proactive strategy. By understanding how different seasons affect your mood, utilizing treatments like light therapy, and making thoughtful adjustments to your lifestyle and medication, you can better manage the symptoms of both SAD and bipolar disorder. This tailored approach should be developed in consultation with your healthcare providers, as this ensures that you can maintain balance and stability, adapting seamlessly as the seasons change.

BIPOLAR DISORDER AND CO-EXISTING HEALTH CONDITIONS

Substance abuse and SAD are not the only disorders to appear alongside bipolar disorder. In fact, there are a variety of comorbidities that can affect the way you manage your bipolar. Whether you are utilizing an integrative care approach or managing it using skills and strategies, it is important to learn how these comorbidities affect one another and how you can treat them.

Common physical and mental health conditions that frequently co-exist with bipolar disorder include cardiovascular diseases, diabetes, and anxiety disorders. Each of these conditions can influence and exacerbate the symptoms of bipolar disorder, creating a complex web of health issues that require careful and coordinated management. It is important to develop a treatment plan alongside your medical team. This confirms your bipolar and comorbidities are both managed. The impact of these co-morbidities on the management of bipolar disorder is significant. This complex interplay between different health conditions necessitates a finely-tuned management plan that considers all aspects of an individual's health (Cuncic, 2024).

An integrated care approach is essential in managing bipolar disorder alongside other co-existing conditions. This approach involves the collaboration of a multidisciplinary team of healthcare providers, including psychiatrists, cardiologists, endocrinologists, and primary care providers, who work together to create a cohesive and comprehensive treatment plan. This plan focuses on treating the symptoms of each condition and minimizing the potential interactions between various treatments and their side effects. It is important for your medical team to be aware of and educate you on the possible complications of treating mental health disorders with a variety of medications (ALTINBAŞ, 2021).

Coordinating care among different healthcare providers is another crucial aspect of managing multiple health conditions. This coordination requires the cooperation of both primary and secondary medical providers, making sure all your healthcare providers are aware of the various aspects of your health and facilitating treatments that are harmonious rather than conflicting. This collaborative approach elevates the quality of care and safeguards treatment adherence, ultimately leading to better health outcomes (Ee et al., 2020).

Effective management also relies heavily on self-management strategies that empower you to take an active role in managing your health. Outside of making a medical treatment plan with your medical team, there are skills you can use to manage your symptoms in the moment before they become second nature. For example, practicing radical acceptance and becoming at peace with your diagnosis can help you prepare for moments when symptoms increase, keeping yourself safe. Practicing awareness of your emotions and reframing negative thoughts also shifts your perspective during times of duress. When applied alongside a medical treatment plan, these skills help you effectively manage your bipolar disorder (Pombo, 2019).

As you steer through the complexities of managing bipolar disorder with other co-existing conditions, remember that comprehensive care is fundamental to achieving stability and maintaining your overall health. From education to medication, there are a variety of strategies and plans to help you manage your bipolar. Through a combination of professional healthcare, self-management, and coordinated care strategies, you can effectively manage the challenges of multiple health conditions, leading to a more balanced and fulfilling life.

LEGAL CONSIDERATIONS: RIGHTS AND RESPONSIBILITIES

Traversing the complexities of bipolar disorder extends beyond medical management and enters the realm of legal rights and responsibilities, a crucial aspect often overshadowed by immediate health concerns. Understanding these legal frameworks is essential, particularly as they pertain to employment and education, where discrimination based on disability can significantly impact your life. Let's learn more about your rights.

In the workplace, the Americans with Disabilities Act (ADA) provides protection against discrimination, promising that individuals with bipolar disorder can request reasonable accommodations to perform their jobs effectively (American Civil Liberties Union, n.d.). Similarly, in educational settings, the ADA requires schools to provide accommodations aimed at leveling the playing field and creating equal educational opportunities. There are protections put in place by the government to verify you can participate in major aspects of life such as work and school. Use online or local resources to educate yourself on your rights (U.S. Department of Education, n.d.).

Navigating insurance systems and healthcare rights can often feel like trying to find your way through a labyrinth, particularly when it comes to mental health services, which are frequently undercovered. Understanding your insurance policy details—what is covered, to what extent, and under what conditions—can make a significant difference in how effectively you manage your disorder, allowing you to make informed decisions about your treatment (National Alliance on Mental Health, n.d.). I have found advocating for yourself in this context involves understanding your rights and learning how to communicate effectively with insurance providers. This might involve preparing detailed documentation of your medical needs, understanding the appeals process for denied claims, and sometimes seeking the help of legal professionals who specialize in health insurance advocacy.

In severe cases of bipolar disorder, legal issues can become particularly complex. Situations may arise where considerations for guardianship, involuntary treatment, or mental health directives need to be addressed. For instance, during severe manic or depressive episodes where an individual's ability to make informed decisions might be impaired, having someone you trust assigned as your guardian can allow you to recover and rest assured that decisions are being made for you in your best interest (Russo Law

Group, P.C., 2024). Similarly, understanding the conditions under which involuntary treatment is considered legally acceptable can help in planning and preventing potential legal conflicts. These legal tools are designed to protect your rights and make sure that treatment decisions are made in your best interest, even when you might not be in a position to express your wishes.

Resources for legal assistance and advocacy play a crucial role in maneuvering through these legal complexities. Organizations such as the National Alliance on Mental Illness (NAMI) offer resources and support for understanding your legal rights and responsibilities. Additionally, legal aid societies, such as the American Bar Association, or disability rights organizations, such as the American Association of People with Disabilities, can provide guidance in legal matters related to disability rights, discrimination, or healthcare coverage. These resources help you advocate for yourself. They empower you to protect your rights effectively, making sure you receive the support and accommodations necessary for managing your condition and addressing any legal matters with confidence.

Understanding and walking in the legal world is a vital component of managing bipolar disorder. By being informed about your rights and utilizing available resources, you can know your legal rights are protected and advocate for your needs. You will rest easier knowing your health management is not hindered by legal or bureaucratic obstacles. This knowledge optimizes your ability to manage your condition and empowers you to advocate for broader changes that can benefit the entire mental health community.

As this chapter concludes, we have explored the special factors that need to be considered when managing bipolar disorder. From educating yourself on potential comorbidities to knowing your legal rights, learning about your condition will benefit you in the long run. In the next chapter, we will learn how valuable empowerment through education is and how knowledge and learning play pivotal roles in managing bipolar disorder and advocating for systemic change.

CHAPTER 7

EMPOWERMENT THROUGH EDUCATION

This chapter is designed to be your compass, guiding you through the complexities of understanding your rights as a patient, advocating for yourself in various medical settings, and maneuvering through the intricacies of healthcare bureaucracy. The information shared here will help you learn to work with the healthcare system with confidence and assertiveness, ensuring that your experience is as smooth and empowered as possible.

UNDERSTANDING YOUR RIGHTS AS A PATIENT

Walking through the healthcare system can often feel like trying to find your way through a mess of information filled with legal jargon and complicated procedures. Yet, understanding your fundamental rights under healthcare laws is crucial. These rights serve as the bedrock of your interactions with healthcare providers.

As a patient with bipolar disorder, you are entitled to the right to informed consent, which means you should be fully informed about the treatments and procedures you are undergoing and consent to them voluntarily, allowing you to decide what is in your best interest. Privacy of your medical information is also paramount. It is guarded under laws like the Health Insurance Portability and Accountability Act (HIPAA), promising your health data is protected and shared only with your consent. Moreover, you have the right to receive a proper standard of care, which means receiving the necessary support from healthcare professionals. Understanding these rights can transform your interactions with the healthcare system from feelings of confusion and helplessness to empowerment and control (Hicks, 2024).

Advocating for oneself in healthcare settings is an essential skill that can significantly affect the outcome of your treatment. It involves speaking up about your needs, questioning treatment plans that do not feel right, and even seeking second opinions when necessary. Effective self-advocacy starts with having a clear understanding of your health condition. This empowers you to engage in informed discussions with your doctors. Prepare for appointments by prioritizing the questions and concerns you may have, perhaps even practicing what you will say beforehand. This preparation helps you make the most of each visit, ensuring that your voice is heard, and your concerns are addressed. Remember, a good healthcare provider will welcome your questions and actively engage with your concerns. If you are unsure of your treatment plan, do not hesitate to ask your medical team questions, potentially seeking a second opinion if needed (Werner, 2023).

Navigating healthcare bureaucracy is another critical aspect of empowering yourself. It involves understanding the ins and outs of health insurance policies, recognizing what is covered, and knowing how to file grievances and appeal denials when necessary. Dealing with insurance can be daunting but understanding your policy details can save you from unexpected medical bills and denied claims. Developing this understanding is a crucial aspect of maximizing your healthcare (BlueCross BlueShield, n.d.). If you encounter issues, most institutions have patient advocates who can help you figure out the complexities of the healthcare system (Coursera, 2023). Additionally, keeping meticulous records of all your interactions, treatments, and correspondence with healthcare providers and insurers can be incredibly beneficial, especially if disputes arise.

Numerous organizations and resources are dedicated to providing support and advocacy for mental health patients. Organizations such as the Substance Abuse and Mental Health Services Administration (SAMHSA) offer a wealth of resources, including providing legal services and investigating rights violations (Substance Abuse and Mental Health Services Administration, n.d.). Additionally, the Depression and Bipolar Support Alliance (DBSA) offers both online and in-person resources that can help you connect with others who understand your condition and are working through similar challenges (Depression and Bipolar Support Alliance, n.d.). Engaging with these resources strengthens your knowledge and advocacy skills. It connects you with a community of support, reinforcing that you are not alone.

Steering through the complexities of the healthcare system with bipolar disorder requires courage, knowledge, and support. By understanding your rights, advocating for your needs, and utilizing available resources, you empower yourself to take control of your health. This empowerment enriches your interactions with healthcare providers, contributing to more effective management of your condition. This leads to better health outcomes and a higher quality of life. As you continue to educate yourself and engage with these tools, remember that each step you take is a step toward greater autonomy and empowerment in your pursuit of the right treatment plan.

EDUCATING FRIENDS AND FAMILY: WORKSHOPS AND RESOURCES

As we've discussed, having a support system is critical to managing your bipolar disorder. With the help of your medical team, friends, and family, you can prepare yourself for triggers and mood episodes. However, it is important for your loved ones to be educated on your condition. There are a variety of ways this can be done. Let's explore them.

The support you receive from friends and family can be refreshing and vital for your recovery and daily management of bipolar disorder. However, the quality of this support often hinges on how well your loved ones understand the condition. Without a solid grasp of what bipolar disorder entails, they may struggle with providing support and compassion. However, with a little bit of education, they can become great resources to help you manage your health and advocate for people with the same condition. This is why it is crucial for your support network to be well-informed—they need to understand not just the clinical facts but the personal experience of living with bipolar disorder (NeuroLaunch, 2023).

Organizing educational sessions can serve as an effective bridge between the knowledge gap that might exist among your friends and family. Consider these sessions as meetings, open, stigma-free spaces where learning meets compassion. You might start by gathering informal, small group discussions at your home or a local space where you can still have privacy. During the meeting, topics can range from understanding the symptoms of bipolar disorder and recognizing the signs of a mood swing to effective ways to offer help during different phases of the cycle. Inviting a healthcare professional or an experienced advocate to speak can add a layer of depth to these discussions, providing expert insights and answering questions that your loved ones may hesitate to ask you directly. It is helpful to have educational materials on hand, such as pamphlets or a short presentation, that attendees can refer to during and after the session. Remember, the goal is to make these sessions as interactive and engaging as possible to maximize understanding and retention of the information.

To further this education outside of the sessions, having a curated list of resources can be invaluable. Books like *An Unquiet Mind* by Kay Redfield Jamison, who herself has bipolar disorder, can offer an intimate glimpse into the life of someone managing the condition. For a more clinical perspective, *The Bipolar Disorder Survival Guide* by David J. Miklowitz provides comprehensive strategies that families can adopt (Boudin, 2023). Online courses offered by platforms like Coursera have courses on mental health that can be accessed easily, providing another layer of understanding through structured, formal education. Articles from reputable sources like the National Institute of Mental Health or Mayo Clinic's website offer up-to-date, research-backed information that can be very useful.

Engagement in community events is another powerful tool in expanding education and reducing stigma. These events provide a broader perspective of the community impacted by bipolar disorder and other mental health conditions, inspiring deeper empathy and understanding. They also offer a chance to meet others who share similar experiences, broadening your support network and providing firsthand insight into how diverse the spectrum of bipolar disorder can be. Attending community events can help you learn to manage symptoms, improving your overall quality of life (Baxter, Burton, and Fancourt, 2022).

Through these educational efforts, friends and family transform from bystanders to allies. They are equipped with understanding and the right tools to offer the support you need. This transformation deepens your relationships, building a community of awareness and sensitivity around bipolar disorder, which is essential for societal change. From educational movies to family events, engaging your loved ones in this way benefits you. It contributes to a larger cultural shift toward acceptance and support for those managing mental health conditions.

ACCESSING AND INTERACTING WITH MEDICAL RESEARCH

Exploring medical research might initially seem daunting, especially when trying to find trustworthy and relevant information about bipolar disorder. Yet, understanding how to access credible sources and interpret their findings is crucial for staying informed about the latest treatments and management strategies, especially when they are strategies that could significantly impact your health and well-being. Each piece of research is a potential tool in your toolkit, something that can empower you to make informed decisions about your treatment options.

The first step is learning how to identify and access reputable medical research sources. Academic journals and professional healthcare websites are foundational elements of quality research. Institutions like public libraries and universities often provide free access to these resources. Websites belonging to established medical institutions like the Mayo Clinic are also valuable sources of up-to-date, research-backed information. When selecting these sources, it is important to check the credentials of the authors and the date of the information to establish whether it is reputable and current or not (University of Washington, n.d.).

Understanding the findings within these research studies is the next critical step. Scientific studies can often be filled with complex terminology and statistical data that might seem impenetrable at first glance. Breaking down a research article starts with understanding its structure, typically composed of an abstract, introduction, methodology, results, and conclusion. Focusing on the introduction (not the abstract) and conclusion can provide a high-level overview of the research and its outcomes (Raff, n.d.).

Staying updated with new studies is vital in a field that progresses as rapidly as mental health treatment. Regularly checking reputable medical journals or organizations that focus on bipolar disorder can provide updates on the latest research. Following influential researchers and professionals on social media platforms like Twitter can also be a strategic move, as many share their latest work and insights online. Additionally, creating a "journal club" with your friends, either virtually or in person, can keep you informed about cutting-edge research, providing opportunities to connect with peers and other individuals who are navigating similar experiences (Rice University, 2020).

Developing critical thinking skills is essential when evaluating the reliability and relevance of research findings and health news. Not all studies are created equal, and some may have biases that could influence their outcomes. Thinking critically and evaluating the sources can help you assess their credibility. Approach things with curiosity and a logical mind. Do not forget to gather information about the source, such as checking if it is peer-reviewed and analyzing the information to determine its credibility (Mind Tools, n.d.).

Being able to evaluate and understand the sources at your disposal helps you check that your bipolar management plan is as effective as it can be. This empowerment through education allows you to engage more confidently with healthcare providers. As you continue to explore and understand the complex world of medical research, remember that each piece of knowledge acquired is a step toward more effective management of your bipolar disorder, contributing to a more informed, healthier life.

THE IMPORTANCE OF ONGOING EDUCATION IN MANAGING BIPOLAR DISORDER

Science is developing at a rapid pace, resulting in better treatment strategies and more information about bipolar disorder. There are plenty of opportunities to continue your education and stay up to date on new developments. Once you have learned the tools and found the resources to help you educate yourself, you will be able to reap the benefits of being an informed patient.

Embracing lifelong learning as a powerful tool for empowerment profoundly changes the way you manage bipolar disorder. From psychoeducation to advocacy, this proactive approach to learning helps you adapt to new treatments, understand evolving medical perspectives, and make informed decisions about your health care. Imagine each piece of new knowledge as a stepping stone that strengthens your path to wellness, allowing you to traverse the complexities of bipolar disorder with increased confidence and competence (MedCircle, n.d.).

Various educational programs, both formal and informal, are available that cater specifically to the needs of those managing chronic conditions like bipolar disorder. Online platforms such as Coursera offer courses on mental health, wellness, and even specific topics like stress management or cognitive-behavioral techniques, as we previously discussed. These courses are often developed by leading experts in the field and provide valuable insights that can be applied directly to daily life. Additionally, many mental health organizations, like the National Alliance on Mental Illness (NAMI), provide resources on health and psychology, which can further develop your understanding and provide you with strategies to manage your condition more effectively.

Engaging in self-education techniques also plays a crucial role in lifelong learning. Personally, I have found setting personal learning goals, for example, can help you stay focused and motivated. Whether it is understanding a new treatment modality, learning a stress-reduction technique, or simply keeping abreast of the latest research, regular education can inform your treatment plan. Keeping a learning journal is another effective strategy. To learn more about journaling with bipolar disorder, see Chapter 5. Additionally, participating in peer learning groups can offer the dual benefits of education and support. These groups can often be found through reputable websites, local community centers and libraries, and your medical team. They offer both learning opportunities and emotional support from others who understand the challenges of living with bipolar disorder. By implementing these things into your day-to-day life, you can continue down your educational path.

The benefits of being an informed patient are manifold and profound. When you actively engage in learning about your health condition, you are better equipped to make informed decisions about your treatment options. You are more likely to choose therapies and interventions that align with your personal health goals and lifestyle, increasing your overall satisfaction. Additionally, an educated approach to managing bipolar disorder significantly increases your satisfaction with healthcare services. Understanding your condition improves your communication with healthcare providers. When you understand the why and how of your treatments, you are more likely to feel in control of your health, which can develop your overall well-being and quality of life (Landmark, 2020).

By embracing ongoing education, you empower yourself with the knowledge and skills needed to manage bipolar disorder confidently. This strengthens your ability to manage your condition effectively, enriching your life. Learning about your disorder helps you make informed decisions and communicate with healthcare providers, increasing overall satisfaction with your treatment plan.

LEVERAGING TECHNOLOGY FOR HEALTH TRACKING AND MANAGEMENT

In an era where technology intertwines seamlessly with daily life, it becomes a pivotal ally in managing health, especially for conditions like bipolar disorder. There are a variety of apps and gadgets that can be used to track steps, nutrition, medication, and doctor's visits. It is possible to incorporate these into your treatment plan as long as it is done safely.

Various apps and digital platforms have been designed to offer more than just convenience. These digital tools function as personal health assistants, helping you keep a detailed log of your daily mental health status. Apps such as Bearable allow you to record your mood, medication intake, and other variables relevant to your condition. This daily tracking helps in identifying patterns or triggers in your mood fluctuations, offering insights that are crucial for the effective management of bipolar disorder.

The utility of these apps extends beyond simple record-keeping. By systematically logging your daily experiences, you create a comprehensive data set that can even better your condition along the way. This information provides real-life snapshots of how your condition manifests over time (Modglin, 20203).

Beyond apps, wearable technology has revolutionized how individuals with bipolar disorder can monitor their health. Devices like the Oura Ring or Apple Watch track physical activity and monitor sleep patterns and heart rate, offering insights into your physical health often correlated with mood changes. The less daunting and personalized nature of these gadgets allows for less daunting approaches to mental health issues. This can be profoundly empowering, allowing for preemptive adjustments in your routine or treatment plan to mitigate these episodes (Busvine, 2024).

Integrating this wealth of data from digital tools into your treatment plans can significantly enrich the care you receive. It allows for a dynamic approach to managing bipolar disorder, where treatment plans are continually refined based on real-time data. The ability to share data with your doctor at the touch of a button allows the doctor to review the detailed data and adjust from there. It educates the patient, giving them a deeper understanding of their body. It transforms a subjective discussion about how you think you have been feeling into an objective, data-driven dialogue about what your numbers are showing. This allows the doctor to see and understand how you do between visits, allowing them to determine if your treatment is effective and tailor your plan accordingly (Rendall, 2023).

While the benefits of using digital tools for health management are substantial, it is crucial to learn the concerns regarding data privacy and security. The personal health information that these apps and devices collect is sensitive. Its protection is paramount. Gadgets like the Oura Ring are in the process of getting a HIPAA-compliant certification (Pastore, 2024). These regulations provide certainty that your data is handled securely and that your privacy is maintained. Always read the privacy policy of any app or device before beginning to use it to understand how your data will be used and who will have access to it. If an app allows, opt for settings that maximize your data privacy, and be cautious about sharing your data. Be proactive about updating your apps and devices to protect against security vulnerabilities. Regular updates often include security patches that can prevent unauthorized access to your data.

Embracing these technologies equips you with powerful tools to manage your bipolar disorder. By integrating these digital solutions into your daily life and treatment planning, you harness the power of data to gain greater control over your condition, ultimately leading to strengthened health outcomes and a better quality of life. Let these tools light your way, providing you with the insights and evidence needed to be an informed and proactive advocate for your health.

PREPARING FOR DOCTOR VISITS AND THERAPY SESSIONS

Navigating your healthcare effectively, especially when dealing with bipolar disorder, requires more than just showing up to your appointments; it demands preparation and active participation. Consider each doctor visit or therapy session as a pivotal meeting where you are not just a patient but an advocate for your health. That knowledge can impart feelings of confidence, knowing you are prepared and ready to tackle your treatment head-on.

To maximize the efficacy of these appointments, begin by preparing a detailed list of symptoms, questions, and topics you wish to discuss. This preparation ensures that no critical information is forgotten. It also helps you steer the conversation toward areas of concern that matter most to you. Documenting your symptoms daily can provide a clear, comprehensive picture of your condition over time. This record is invaluable during your appointments as it provides concrete data to your healthcare provider, facilitating a more tailored treatment approach. Consider bringing someone with you as support, especially if you need assistance with notetaking or remembering important things (IDCC Health Services, 2023).

Effective communication is the cornerstone of these interactions. It involves more than the ability to speak—it is about making sure you are heard and understood. Begin by engaging in active communication, using honesty as a foundation, and sharing your experience openly. Active listening is also important. Listen carefully to your medical provider. If a treatment plan sounds confusing or overwhelming, it is crucial to ask for clarification until you fully understand the information provided. Remember, the goal of these sessions is not just to receive care but to engage in a collaborative process that respects your views and preferences (IDCC Health Services, 2023).

Documenting and tracking your progress through health journals or apps is more than a task—it is an empowerment tool. It allows you to monitor your health, understand patterns, and recognize achievements, no matter how small. Collect your symptoms and mood tracking with your questions and concerns, keeping them all in one place. Bring this journal to your appointments to help create a more dynamic and informed dialogue with your healthcare provider. This practice helps make necessary adjustments to your treatment plans by collecting critical information. It also celebrates progress, which can be incredibly motivating (IDCC Health Services, 2023).

Follow-up and action plans are critical in maintaining the continuity of care. Before leaving any appointment, make sure you have a clear understanding of any new treatment suggestions, including changes to medication or lifestyle adjustments. Discuss how to integrate these into your daily routine, requesting alternative options if you are unhappy with the plan. Clarify any follow-up appointments to check your progress. Keep a dedicated section in your health journal for follow-up notes, which can guide your preparation for the next appointment, promising each meeting builds on the last, moving you steadily toward your health goals.

As you step forward from this section, equipped with strategies to prepare, communicate, document, and follow up, you hold the keys to turning every doctor visit and therapy session into a step toward better health management. Engaging actively in these sessions positively impacts your treatment outcome and deepens your understanding of your condition, supporting a sense of control and confidence.

As we close this chapter, carry forward the understanding that your proactive involvement is crucial in dealing with the complexities of bipolar disorder, and each interaction with healthcare providers is an opportunity to advocate for a better quality of life. Let this empowerment through active participation be your guide as you continue to explore and adopt further strategies for managing your condition in the following chapters.

CHAPTER 8

LIVING A FULFILLING LIFE WITH BIPOLAR DISORDER

This chapter is dedicated to illuminating paths that others have walked, turning their challenges into victories, and drawing a map for you to find and celebrate your own successes. Each narrative shared here is not just a story; it is a beacon of hope, a testament to the resilience of the human spirit, and a proof that stability and success are within reach, regardless of the hurdles bipolar disorder places in your path.

SUCCESS STORIES: REAL-LIFE EXAMPLES OF OVERCOMING CHALLENGES

When living with bipolar disorder, nothing is more empowering than real-life examples of individuals who have managed their condition and carved out successful and fulfilling lives. These stories serve as a lighthouse, guiding you through stormy waters to potential harbors of success and stability.

Take, for instance, the story of Tracye, who was diagnosed with bipolar during her college years. It was a challenging diagnosis.

She was only familiar with stereotypes and stigma surrounding bipolar disorder. Her twenties were difficult as she struggled with the disorder without medication. She managed to survive, graduating college and securing a good job, but her bipolar still was not being treated, and it was affecting her deeply. During hypomanic and manic episodes, she partied hard, spending more money than she had and entering into toxic relationships. It all came to a boiling point in the fall of 2017 when she finally broke down due to the stressors of life and decided to seek help. Her struggle with medication and bipolar disorder ultimately led to her losing her job, friends, and almost her family. After four months of struggling with medication, she finally started to come out on top, ultimately discovering a better life. Her life and experience stand as a story of recovery and hope (Bergeron, 2021).

From Tracye's story, several key strategies emerge that you can apply to your own life. First, the importance of a tailored treatment plan cannot be overstressed—each person is unique, and their treatment plans should be the same way. Finding the right combination of medication, therapy, and lifestyle changes is crucial. Second, the role of support systems—both professional and personal—plays a critical role in managing bipolar disorder. Knowing you have people, whether they are friends or family, who understand and support you can make a significant difference in your recovery and ongoing management (Bergeron, 2021).

Moreover, this narrative, and others like it, underlines the importance of resilience and hope. Each individual's story highlights the necessity of consistent effort—adjusting strategies as needed and educating yourself on the reality of bipolar disorder so you can challenge them as needed. This consistent effort often leads to substantial improvements in quality of life, enabling individuals to manage their condition effectively and thrive (Bergeron, 2021).

It is important to recognize that managing bipolar disorder is not a sprint but a marathon. Small, daily victories accumulate over time, leading to significant long-term success. Creating a routine, practicing self-compassion, and tracking progress are all part of the dynamic process of living with bipolar disorder. Consistency is crucial to getting mentally and emotionally healthier (Zrpath Behavioral Health Services, 2023).

Each story of success serves as a testament to individual resilience. It is an inspiration for adapting to your circumstances. Whether it is finding the right medication regimen, discovering the therapeutic power of a hobby, or leveraging the support of loved ones, the paths to managing bipolar disorder are as diverse as they are hopeful. As you reflect on these stories, consider how the lessons learned might be incorporated into your own life, helping you to build a resilient, fulfilling life despite the challenges posed by bipolar disorder.

MAINTAINING LONG-TERM RELATIONSHIPS WHILE MANAGING BIPOLAR DISORDER

Relationships are complicated even without juggling a mental illness. With bipolar disorder, it takes on a different kind of complexity. Communicating, compromising, and building a relationship on support and trust provides you with the tools to create a thriving relationship.

Open and honest dialogue is not just beneficial but essential in facilitating understanding and managing expectations between you and your loved ones. Consider the dynamics in any relationship. Misunderstandings can escalate into conflicts when feelings or expectations are not clearly expressed or understood. For someone living with bipolar disorder, where emotions can be particularly intense and sometimes unpredictable, the stakes are even higher. Effective communication involves expressing your feelings honestly, such as being open about your diagnosis. It also means keeping an open line of communication, being open with them rather than expecting them to read your mind. This helps in adjusting expectations and provides a platform for mutual understanding and support, which is crucial during both stable periods and episodes of mood swings (Cirino, 2024).

Living with bipolar disorder might sometimes require you to prioritize your health needs, such as attending therapy sessions, maintaining a strict medication schedule, or needing space during mood swings. While it is crucial to balance these needs with your obligations and roles in your relationships, you need to make sure you are cared for first. Otherwise, you will not be able to care for your partner. This balance between caring for yourself and your partner creates space for your relationship to remain strong and supportive rather than becoming another source of stress (Bailey, 2018). It involves practical steps like planning ahead for mood fluctuations, involving your partner in your health management plan, and setting aside quality time to spend together (Cirino, 2024). Verifying neither your health needs nor your relationship obligations are neglected helps you develop a supportive and enduring relationship.

Support from partners can significantly influence the management of bipolar disorder. Partners can play various roles—from supporting you day-to-day to helping you manage mood episodes and attending therapy sessions. However, their involvement does not always need to be serious. Sometimes, taking part in fun and beneficial activities like exercise or enjoying symptom-free times can bring light into the relationship. Encouraging your partner to be informed about bipolar disorder can develop their ability to support you effectively. This shared responsibility eases your burden, strengthening the bond between you and your partner, making it a true partnership in every sense (Martin, 2021).

Building and maintaining trust with your partner is crucial in any relationship, but it is especially significant when one partner is managing a condition like bipolar disorder. Trust is built through consistent behavior, reliability, and mutual respect—qualities that reassure both partners of their commitment to each other. Reliability can be shown in small, everyday actions—being on time, following through on commitments, or just being there when you say you will be. These actions demonstrate to your partner that they can rely on you, proving that your words and actions are aligned and reinforcing trust. Mutual respect involves acknowledging each other's needs, boundaries, and contributions to the relationship. It means clearly and honestly communicating your expectations and feelings, and it is essential for maintaining a healthy and supportive relationship. Together, these elements create a strong foundation of trust that can withstand the challenges that come with managing bipolar disorder, making sure the relationship survives and thrives (P. Abigail, 2024).

In cultivating these aspects of your relationships, remember that small, consistent efforts can lead to significant, lasting impacts. Whether it is through improving communication or building trust, each step you take strengthens your ability to maintain fulfilling and supportive relationships. These relationships, in turn, provide a vital network of support that can enrich your quality of life and your ability to manage bipolar disorder effectively, allowing you to enjoy your loved ones.

CAREER PLANNING AND PROGRESSION WITH BIPOLAR DISORDER

Just like relationships, choosing and maintaining a career while managing bipolar disorder can be difficult. From choosing a career and advancing in it to deciding whether to disclose or not, there is a lot to consider. It is important to find a balance between caring for yourself and thriving in your career.

Traversing the professional world with bipolar disorder involves a nuanced approach to career planning, where considerations include how well a position accommodates the realities of your condition. Choosing a career or a specific job involves evaluating several critical factors, such as the workplace environment, which can add to stress levels typically associated with the role and the flexibility of the schedule. For instance, a more competitive workplace may have rigid schedules or an increase in stress, which might pose challenges. Roles that allow for flexible working hours and provide a supportive, understanding environment can significantly optimize your ability to manage your condition effectively (Bowman, n.d.).

Advancing in your career while managing bipolar disorder requires dedication to your role and strategic planning around your health management. Developing a robust personal system for stress management is crucial. This might involve things we have previously discussed, such as regular check-ins with a mental health professional, using stress-reduction techniques such as mindfulness or meditation during breaks, and establishing a support network of colleagues or a mentor within the workplace who understands your condition and can offer support when needed. A structured workplace can help reduce stress and, as a result, reduce potential triggers. It is also helpful to develop new skills periodically, keeping your mind agile and making you a more appealing employee. When deciding what skills to learn, consider developing short- and long-term goals to help guide you (Bowman, n.d.).

The question of whether to disclose your bipolar disorder at work is complex and deeply personal. As we discussed in Chapter 4, there are things to consider when deciding whether or not to disclose your condition to your employer. If you choose to disclose, it is advisable to do it in a controlled and planned manner, perhaps starting with a trusted HR representative or a direct supervisor who has shown understanding and supportiveness in matters of employee health. It is also beneficial to be informed about your legal rights under employment law, which can protect you from discrimination based on your condition (Seven, 2023).

Success stories abound of individuals who have managed their bipolar disorder successfully within their careers. They used their experiences to cultivate environments of greater understanding and support for others with similar conditions, helping to reduce stigma and further their career. Consider the example of a corporate executive. After disclosing her condition, she worked with her HR department to establish a series of mental health workshops that educated her colleagues about bipolar disorder and other mental health issues. This helped inspire a more supportive workplace culture. Another example is a teacher who, by carefully managing his schedule and stress levels, utilized his experiences with bipolar disorder to connect with and support students dealing with similar challenges. In doing so, he advanced his effectiveness as an educator and advocate.

These stories highlight the potential for success and the importance of strategic planning, self-awareness, and advocacy in guiding one's career while managing bipolar disorder. As you consider your own career path, remember your experiences with bipolar disorder provide you with unique insights and strengths that can enrich your professional life and offer valuable perspectives to your colleagues and industry. With the right approach, you can succeed professionally, contributing positively to making the workplace a more inclusive and supportive environment.

LONG-TERM FINANCIAL PLANNING AND STABILITY

Managing finances can be difficult even without bipolar disorder. When you are facing challenges like mania, which can result in irresponsible spending, it is important to identify potential challenges that may impact your budget and protect your assets. On top of that, you will need to consider the healthcare costs required to help you manage your bipolar. Let's explore these topics further, starting with identifying financial challenges.

Managing finances effectively poses a unique set of challenges when you are living with bipolar disorder. The condition can lead to impulsive spending during manic phases and periods of financial neglect during depressive episodes. These challenges can lead to struggling with debt unless there is an active effort made to protect your budget and assets. Recognizing these potential hurdles is the first step toward crafting a strategy that safeguards your financial health and protects long-term stability (Moezzi, 2023).

The cornerstone of sound financial management, particularly for someone managing bipolar disorder, is a well-structured budget. Creating and adhering to a budget helps maintain control over your finances, reducing stress that could trigger mood episodes. Begin by tracking your income and expenses to understand where your money goes each month. Do your best to be honest about it so you have a clear picture of how much you make and spend. This might seem daunting at first, but using tools like autopay and direct deposit features can do some of the work for you. These tools help verify bills are being paid. This is especially useful during depressive episodes when such tasks can feel overwhelming. It is also wise to include savings in your budget as a regular expense item, which can build a financial cushion and offer peace of mind during periods of reduced income or unexpected expenses. Do not be afraid to rely on your support system and ask for help when you need it (Moezzie, 2023).

Planning for healthcare costs is another critical aspect that requires attention. Bipolar disorder often involves ongoing expenses such as medications, therapy sessions, and sometimes hospitalization, which can add up significantly over time. Start by thoroughly understanding your health insurance coverage—know what treatments and medications are covered and to what extent. It is important to understand what your premium and deductible are and how much you will end up paying out of pocket. This can be factored into your budget once you have identified your income and spending (Centers for Medicare and Medicaid Services, n.d.). For medications, look into patient assistance programs offered by pharmaceutical companies or reputable online sources. You should also talk to your doctor about alternatives that may save you money (Davis, 2023).

Protecting your assets during periods of mood instability is also crucial. Legal instruments such as a financial power of attorney can be invaluable during times when you might not have the capacity to manage your finances effectively. In times of duress, such as during manic or depressive episodes, this can help confirm your assets are safe. Setting up trusts can also be a strategic way to manage and protect larger assets. When working with a trusted company, try to find one that is experienced in dealing with health issues (Swingle, 2024).

Embracing these strategies helps in mitigating the financial challenges associated with bipolar disorder. It empowers you to build and maintain financial stability. Regular reviews of your financial plan, ideally with a financial advisor who understands your situation, can verify your strategies remain aligned with your changing needs and circumstances. By taking proactive steps toward financial management, you are securing your economic future and contributing positively to your overall well-being and peace of mind, allowing you to focus more on managing your health and less on financial stress.

TRAVEL AND LEISURE: ENJOYING LIFE RESPONSIBLY

Going on travel adventures or indulging in leisure activities can seem daunting when you are managing bipolar disorder, yet these experiences are not just possible—they're also potentially enriching and therapeutic. In this section, we will discuss planning for travel, how you can incorporate travel for your mental health, potential risks, and how to manage them. You will find examples of individuals who have successfully enjoyed traveling with bipolar disorder. Let's get started.

The key lies in thoughtful preparation that accommodates your health needs, making sure your adventures are not just safe but also enjoyable. It is essential to consult with your healthcare provider about your travel plans and assess whether you are in a stable phase. They can offer guidance tailored to your condition, which might include letting them know about your travel plans and sharing your itinerary (Brown, 2021). This can be helpful in identifying potential overstimulation and triggers. They will also be able to review your medication plan to ensure you will be covered and not run out.

The importance of incorporating leisure and relaxation into your routine cannot be overstated. Leisure activities can have significant therapeutic effects. Simply reading in a quiet park can significantly reduce stress and better your overall mood. These activities provide a break from the routine and offer a sense of peace and rejuvenation. They are not just fillers in your schedule; they are vital practices that help maintain your mental health, serving as a counterbalance to the pressures and routines of daily life. Make sure you have a plan B, just in case you need to make adjustments for your mental health (Flanigan, 2023)

Managing risks while traveling is also paramount. There are a variety of potential triggers that come with breaking your routine. For example, disrupting your sleep routine and experiencing jet lag can influence your mood and potentially cause an episode. Having a clear plan for what to do if you experience a mood episode away from home is crucial. Part of this is having a conversation with your medical and support teams. They can help you plan your medication and coping skills and prepare for potentially experiencing worse symptoms than usual. This preparation will prepare you so that wherever you are, you have a safety net that can support you if needed (Brown, 2021).

Real-life stories of individuals with bipolar disorder who have successfully managed their condition while traveling can be incredibly inspiring. Let's take a look at Andrea, a mother with bipolar disorder. She traveled between Asia and the United States, finding it stressful, especially while managing her mental health. She was careful to make sure she had the medication she needed, avoiding mishaps, and focused on the positives, like quality time with her family. Ultimately, she found things like lavender oil and healthy exercise helped manage the stress (Brankin, 2024).

As you consider incorporating more travel and leisure into your life, remember that these activities are not just possible; they are also beneficial. They provide a vital opportunity to relax, recharge, and experience the world through a new lens, all while managing your health responsibly. The key is to plan thoughtfully and embrace the experiences that bring you joy and peace. With proper preparation and support, you can enjoy your vacation to the fullest.

SETTING AND ACHIEVING PERSONAL GOALS DESPITE BIPOLAR DISORDER

Living with bipolar disorder often requires not just managing the condition itself but also maintaining a clear vision of your aspirations and goals. There are tips and tricks to setting and achieving goals when you are dealing with bipolar disorder. Special techniques to help you set goals that work for you and focus on them will have you celebrating milestones in no time. The first thing to do is determine what your goals are.

Goal setting, when done thoughtfully, can be a powerful process that brings structure and motivation to your life, turning aspirations into tangible achievements. Embracing the S.M.A.R.T (Specific, Measurable, Achievable, Relevant, Time-bound) criteria in setting your goals ensures they are well-defined, realistic, and within reach, even amidst the challenges posed by bipolar disorder. When setting goals, it is crucial to tailor them specifically to your situation, taking into account the variability of your condition. Begin by defining specific outcomes you want to achieve, which can range from completing a short course to launching a small business. Confirm these goals are measurable, such as setting milestones you can track. It is important that these goals are achievable. Each goal should be relevant to your broader life ambitions. Finally, establish a clear timeline for each goal to provide structure and urgency, keeping in mind the need for flexibility should your health requirements change (Mind Tools, n.d.).

Staying motivated and maintaining focus can be particularly challenging during periods when your mood affects your energy and outlook. Strategies to increase motivation might include finding what motivates you, such as incentives or rewards, and utilizing that. Even writing your goals down can help solidify them and create a plan for achieving them. Set up small, daily tasks that contribute to a larger goal, providing a sense of accomplishment regularly. During times when motivation wanes, try to visualize the end results, giving you a boost to keep going and ultimately reach your goals (Indeed, 2023).

Celebrating milestones is crucial in maintaining morale and motivation. Each milestone achieved is a step toward your larger goal. Make it a habit to acknowledge and celebrate these achievements, however small they may seem, as they positively reinforce the good behaviors and attitudes that got you there. This could be as simple as treating yourself to a favorite meal, sharing your progress with friends or family, or taking a well-deserved break. These celebrations reinforce positive feelings and can increase your motivation to pursue the next milestone (Maryville University, 2021).

Adjusting your goals as your treatment progresses and your personal circumstances develop is also essential. Bipolar disorder can be unpredictable, and what may seem achievable at one time can become daunting at another time. Do not hesitate to refine or even overhaul your goals if they no longer fit your life path or if they become too overwhelming. Adjusting goals is not a sign of failure but a sign of your ability to adapt and grow. This flexibility allows you to stay committed to your overall growth without being tied down to objectives that no longer serve you (Brennan, 2023).

Remember, the process of setting and pursuing goals is just as important as the outcome. Each step you take builds skills, confidence, and resilience, allowing you to manage bipolar disorder with strength and grace. By setting realistic, well-structured goals and adapting them as you grow, you grow your ability to manage your condition, empowering yourself to lead a fulfilling and productive life.

In this chapter, we explored living life successfully with bipolar disorder. Hearing success stories from others gives hope that things can always get better. When taking a look at the challenges people with bipolar face, you can begin to find solutions and ways to explore the challenges of the world. From maintaining long-term relationships to planning and progressing in your career, you can live a fulfilling life complete with financial stability and time for leisure and travel.

A CHANCE TO EMPOWER OTHERS

As you move forward on your journey with strength and determination, take a moment to offer the same opportunity to others.

Simply by sharing your honest opinion of this book and a little about what you've gained from it, you'll help other people navigating the complexities of bipolar disorder to find the guidance they're looking for.

WANT TO HELP OTHERS?

Thank you so much for your support. You're making a huge difference.

Scan the QR code below:

CONCLUSION

From our initial steps in understanding the nuances of bipolar disorder, through the intricate paths of managing daily life, treatments, and support systems, to empowering yourself through continuous education and embracing a fulfilling life, our expedition has been rich and enlightening. Navigating bipolar disorder can be daunting without the right resources. The hope is that you find a compass in this book and, in conjunction with your medical provider, can use it to manage your mental health effectively.

We began by decoding the complexities of bipolar disorder, stressing the importance of an accurate diagnosis and personalized management and treatment strategies. Taking into consideration factors like support systems, workplace dynamics, and coping mechanisms, you can start to see how you are not alone in your experience and have the support and help you need to be successful. Educating yourself on the disorder and the special considerations when dealing with bipolar can help you live a fulfilling life. Each chapter built upon the last, combining strategies and insights: the support of loved ones, the empowerment that comes from informed education, and the unveiling of a life filled with potential despite the challenges posed by bipolar disorder.

A recurring theme in our discussions has been the power of hope and resilience when it comes to your life with bipolar disorder. Do not forget that with the right strategies, a robust support system, and an informed understanding, achieving a stable and rewarding life with bipolar disorder is possible. You are encouraged to continue educating yourself, staying abreast of the latest research, and advocating for yourself and others within the bipolar community.

Take charge of your health with the proactive management strategies we have explored. Embrace self-care diligently, finding methods of practicing mindfulness. Adhere to your treatment plans and utilize the coping mechanisms that work best for you, helping you keep your bipolar under control. Remember the strength that lies in a supportive community. Whether it is healthcare providers, family, friends, or support groups, the value of a nurturing network cannot be overstated. Do not forget to flip back through the book, reviewing sections as needed to help you stay on track.

Bipolar disorder presents its challenges—moments of uncertainty and days of struggle. Yet, within these challenges lie opportunities for immense growth and profound self-discovery. Approach each day with the knowledge that the potential for living a rich and meaningful life is well within your reach. Know that you are doing the work to get where you want to, and it will be worth it in the long run. You are resilient and capable of managing your mental health with care and grace.

I want to thank you sincerely for your trust and time while going on this journey with me. It is my hope that this book serves as a guide and a source of comfort and strength. Let it stand as a reminder that you are not alone in this. You are part of a community, a collective that understands, supports, and uplifts each other.

Let us move forward with a message of empowerment. You are equipped to manage the complexities of bipolar disorder with compassion and strength. Continue to share your stories, reach out for help when needed, and contribute to breaking down the stigmas associated with mental health.

I stand with you. Together, let us continue to strive toward a life not defined by bipolar disorder but enriched by the depth it adds to our experiences and the strength it calls forth from within us.

REFERENCES

Ackerman, Courtney E. 2017. "CBT Techniques: 25 Cognitive Behavioral Therapy Worksheets." Published March 20, 2017. https://positivepsychology.com/cbt-cognitive-behavioral-therapy-techniques-worksheets/#cbt-tools

Ackerman, Courtney E. 2018. "Cognitive Restructuring Techniques for Reframing Thoughts." Published February 12, 2018. https://positivepsychology.com/cbt-cognitive-restructuring-cognitive-distortions/#hero-single

Aldinger, Fanny, and Thomas G. Schulze. 2017. "Environmental Factors, Life Events, and Trauma in the Course of Bipolar Disorder." *Psychiatry and Clinical Neurosciences* 71 (1): 6–17. doi:10.1111/pcn.12433.

ALTINBAŞ, Kürşat. 2021. "Treatment of Comorbid Psychiatric Disorders with Bipolar Disorder." *Archives of Neuropsychiatry* 58 (Suppl 1): S41–46. doi:10.29399/npa.27615.

American Civil Liberties Union. n.d. "Disability Rights." Accessed July 9, 2024. https://www.aclu.org/know-your-rights/disability-rights

American Psychiatric Association. n.d. "Stigma, Prejudice and Discrimination Against People with Mental Illness." Accessed July 3, 2024. https://www.psychiatry.org/patients-families/stigma-and-discrimination

American Psychiatric Association. n.d. "What is Cognitive Behavioral Therapy?" Accessed July 5, 2024. https://www.apa.org/ptsd-guideline/patients-and-families/cognitive-behavioral

Anderson, Katy. 2023. "Why You Should Take Medication as Subscribed." Last modified July 25, 2023. https://www.singlecare.com/blog/medication-adherence/

Association for Behavioral and Cognitive Therapies. n.d. "Treatment Options: CBT or Medication." Accessed July 7, 2024. https://www.abct.org/get-help/treatment-options-cbt-or-medication/

Badosa, Hector. n.d. "Daily Delights: Exploring Hobbies and Activities of Daily Living." Accessed July 5, 2024. https://hobbiesblog.com/hobbies-and-activities-of-daily-living/

Bailey, Eileen. 2018. "9 Rules for Bipolar Relationships." Last modified June 12, 2018. https://www.healthcentral.com/slideshow/9-rules-for-bipolar-relationships

Brankin, Andrea McKenna. 2024. "I Have an Invisible Disability. Flying is Extra Stressful, and Other Travelers Don't Understand Why." Published March 11,

2024. https://www.businessinsider.com/mom-with-disability-bipolar-disorder-travel-abroad-stress-medication-2024-3

Brennan. 2023. "Goals Are Meant to be Adjusted: Here is How." Published June 21, 2023. https://hypercontext.com/blog/work-goals/goals-are-meant-to-be-adjusted-here-is-how

Baxter, Louise, Alexandra Burton, and Daisy Fancourt. 2022. "Community and Cultural Engagement for People with Lived Experience of Mental Health Conditions: What Are the Barriers and Enablers?" *BMC Psychology* 10 (1): 71. doi:10.1186/s40359-022-00775-y.

Beasley, Elizabeth. 2021. "Best Hobbies for Mental Health." Last modified March 29, 2021. https://www.healthgrades.com/right-care/mental-health-and-behavior/best-hobbies-for-mental-health

Bedosky, Lauren. 2024. "How to Journal: A Detailed Beginner's Guide to Therapeutic Writing and Drawing." Last modified March 2, 2024. https://www.everydayhealth.com/emotional-health/how-to-journal-a-detailed-beginners-guide/

Bergeron, Tracye. 2021. "Living with Bipolar Disorder: Tracye's Story." Published July 9, 2021. https://www.healthline.com/health/bipolar-disorder/bipolar-pov

Blackwell, Caira. 2023. "The Best Meditation Apps." Last modified November 15, 2023. https://www.nytimes.com/wirecutter/reviews/best-meditation-apps/

BlueCross BlueShield. n.d. "Understanding Heath Coverage to Maximize Your Care." Accessed July 10, 2024. https://www.bcbs.com/the-health-of-america/articles/understanding-health-insurance-coverage-maximize-your-care

Borenstein, Jeffrey. 2020. "Distinguishing Bipolar Disorder from Major Depression." Published May 11, 2020. https://www.psychologytoday.com/us/blog/brain-and-behavior/202005/distinguishing-bipolar-disorder-major-depression

Boudin, Melissa. 2023. "25 Best Books About Bipolar Disorder." Published May 9, 2023. https://www.choosingtherapy.com/books-on-bipolar/

Bowman, Sam. n.d. "Navigating the Work World as a Person with Bipolar Disorder." Accessed July 12, 2024. https://ibpf.org/navigating-the-work-world-as-a-person-with-bipolar-disorder/

Bowman, Sam. n.d. "Supporting Career Development for Individuals with Bipolar Disorder: Online Resources and Job Search Strategies." Accessed July 12, 2024. https://ibpf.org/supporting-career-development-for-individuals-with-bipolar-disorder-online-resources-and-job-search-strategies/

Bradley, John. 2023. "The Art of Embracing Failure: Learning and Growing from Setbacks." Published July 9, 2023. https://medium.com/lampshade-of-illumination/the-art-of-embracing-failure-learning-and-growing-from-setbacks-af7a6dbe6b5c

Bressert, Steve. 2021. "What Causes Bipolar Disorder." Last modified February 11, 2021. https://psychcentral.com/bipolar/bipolar-disorder-causes

Brown, Madelyn. 2021. "8 Ways to Fully Benefit from Travel for Folks with Bipolar Disorder." Last modified November 9, 2021. https://psychcentral.com/bipolar/travel-tips-for-people-with-bipolar-disorder

Busvine, Alice. 2024. "Top 10 Mental Health Wearables and Gadgets." Published January 30, 2024. https://techround.co.uk/tech/mental-health-wearables-gadgets/#:~:text=Apple%20Watch,improvement%20for%20their%20mental%20health.

Casabianca, Sandra Silva. 2021. "Coping with Bipolar Disorders: 5 Self-Help Strategies." Last modified January 18, 2021. https://psychcentral.com/lib/self-help-strategies-for-bipolar-disorder

Centers for Medicare and Medicaid Services. n.d. "Manage Your Health Care Costs." Accessed July 13, 2024. https://www.cms.gov/about-cms/agency-information/omh/downloads/c2c-manage-your-healthcare-costs-508.pdf

Cherney, Kristeen. 2019. "What You Should Know About Bipolar Disorder and Pregnancy." Published October 19, 2017. https://www.healthline.com/health/bipolar-disorder/bipolar-pregnancy

Cherry, Kendra. 2022. "Benefits of Mindfulness." Last modified September 2, 2022. https://www.verywellmind.com/the-benefits-of-mindfulness-5205137

Cherry, Kendra. 2023. "Why Work-Life Balance is so Important—and How to Nail It." Published October 21, 2023. https://www.verywellmind.com/why-work-life-balance-is-so-important-8374683

Cirino, Erica. 2024. "Guide to Bipolar Disorder and Relationships." Last modified February 8, 2024. https://www.healthline.com/health/bipolar-disorder/relationship-guide

Clarke, Jodi. 2021. "Healthy Ways to Celebrate Success." Last modified October 7, 2021. https://www.verywellmind.com/healthy-ways-to-celebrate-success-4163887

Clear Mind Treatment. 2024. "Unveiling the Power of Holistic and Alternative Treatments for Bipolar Disorder in Los Angeles." Published July 15, 2024. https://clearmindtreatment.com/blog/unveiling-the-power-of-holistic-and-alternative-treatments-for-bipolar-disorder-in-los-angeles/

Cleveland Clinic. n.d. "Mood Stabilizers." Accessed July 5, 2024. https://my.clevelandclinic.org/health/articles/mood-stabilizers

Cohen, Ilene Strauss. 2024. "Setting Firm and Consistent Boundaries with Your Family." Published January 2, 2024. https://www.psychologytoday.com/us/blog/your-emotional-meter/202401/setting-firm-and-consistent-boundaries-with-your-family

Cohut, Maria. 2018. "What are the Benefits of Being Creative?" Published February

16, 2018. https://www.medicalnewstoday.com/articles/320947#_noHeaderPrefixedContent

Coursera. 2023. "What is a Patient Advocate? (And What Do They Do)" Last modified November 29, 2023. https://www.coursera.org/articles/patient-advocate

Cox, Janelle. 2023. "How are Seasonal Patterns Related to Bipolar Disorder?" Published February 9, 2023. https://psychcentral.com/bipolar/seasonal-bipolar

Crider, Catherine. 2023. "How to Use a Symptoms Journal." Published July 25, 2023. https://www.healthline.com/health/symptoms-journal

Cuncic, Arlin. 2024. "Comorbidities in Mental Health." Last modified April 8, 2024. https://www.verywellmind.com/what-is-comorbidity-3024480

Currin-Sheehan, Kristen. 2021. "Rinse, Repeat. Besting Bipolar Disorder with Routines." Last modified February 19, 2021. https://psychcentral.com/bipolar/building-a-routine-when-you-have-bipolar-disorder#creating-a-routine

Currin-Sheehan, Kristin and Elaina J. Martin. 2021. "Popular Vitamins for Bipolar Disorder." Last modified April 28, 2021. https://psychcentral.com/bipolar/vitamins-for-bipolar-disorder

Davies, Nicola. 2020. "Advances in Psychiatry Biomarkers." Published November 5, 2020. https://www.psychiatryadvisor.com/news/advances-in-psychiatry-biomarkers/

Davis, Julie. 2023. "How to Save Money on Prescriptions." Published November 21, 2023. https://www.webmd.com/health-insurance/ss/slideshow-money-saving-tips-drug-costs

Depression and Bipolar Support Alliance. n.d. "Support." Accessed July 10, 2024. https://www.dbsalliance.org/support/

DiPirro, Dani. 2020. "6 Self-Care Tips for the Changing Seasons." Published November 12, 2020. https://welldoing.org/article/6-self-care-tips-changing-seasons

Ee, C., J. Lake, J. Firth, F. Hargraves, M. de Manincor, T. Meade, W. Marx, and J. Sarris. 2020. "An Integrative Collaborative Care Model for People with Mental Illness and Physical Comorbidities." *International Journal of Mental Health Systems* 14 (November): 83. doi:10.1186/s13033-020-00410-6.

Eisenstadt, Leah, 2022. "Researchers Find First Strong Genetic Risk Factor for Bipolar Disorder." Published April 6, 2022. https://www.broadinstitute.org/news/researchers-find-first-strong-genetic-risk-factor-bipolar-disorder

Ellie Mental Health. 2023. "The Synergy of Therapy and Medication: Enhancing Mental Health Treatment." Published August 23, 2023. https://elliementalhealth.com/the-synergy-of-therapy-and-medication-enhancing-mental-health-treatment/

Etcheson, Serena. 2021. "The Importance of Educating Family Members about

Mental Health." Published August 1, 2021. https://www.stepupformentalhealth.org/the-importance-of-educating-family-members-about-mental-health/

Fabbri, Chiara. 2021. "The Role of Genetics in Bipolar Disorder." *Current Topics in Behavioral Neurosciences* 48: 41–60. doi:10.1007/7854_2020_153.

Faulkner, Rod T. 2023. "How Reviewing Old Journal Entries Can Fuel Personal Growth." Published November 4, 2023. https://medium.com/free-thinkr/how-reviewing-old-journal-entries-can-fuel-personal-growth-d898fb7e33da

Ferguson, Sian. 2021. "What's the Difference Between BPD and Bipolar Disorder?" Published May 11, 2021. https://psychcentral.com/disorders/bpd-vs-bipolar-disorder

Flanigan, Robin L. 2023. "Balancing Your Vacation with Bipolar Disorder." Last modified June 2, 2023. https://www.bphope.com/balancing-your-vacation-with-bipolar-disorder/

Fletcher, Jenna. 2023. "What to Know about Bipolar II Disorder." Last modified October 25, 2023. https://www.medicalnewstoday.com/articles/319280

Forbes Technology Council. 2019. "A Beginner's Guide to Online Privacy: 12 Important Tips. Published June 7, 2019. https://www.forbes.com/sites/forbestechcouncil/2019/06/07/a-beginners-guide-to-online-privacy-12-important-tips/

Gillette, Hope. 2023. "9 Triggers for Bipolar I Disorder Mood Episodes and How to Manage Them." Published January 26, 2023. https://www.healthline.com/health/bipolar-disorder/bipolar-mood-episode-triggers#managing-triggers

Ginta, Daniela. 2022. "Bipolar Disorder and Schizophrenia: What Are the Differences?" Last modified June 23, 2022. https://www.healthline.com/health/bipolar-disorder/bipolar-vs-schizophrenia

Gold, Alexandra. 2022. "Activity Scheduling for Bipolar Depression." Published October 2, 2022. https://www.psychologytoday.com/us/blog/living-well-bipolar-disorder/202210/activity-scheduling-bipolar-depression

Grey, Heather. 2024. "9 Myths and Facts About Bipolar Disorder You Should Know." Published January 3, 2024. https://www.healthline.com/health/bipolar-disorder/myths-and-facts-about-bipolar

Grey, Heather. 2023. "Your FAQs Around How to Live with Someone Who Has Bipolar Disorder." Last modified July 25, 2023. https://psychcentral.com/bipolar/living-with-someone-who-has-bipolar-disorder

Gurarie, Mark. 2024. "Why Does Bipolar Disorder Get Worse with Age?" Last modified March 4, 2024. https://www.verywellhealth.com/does-bipolar-get-worse-with-age-8548441#toc-how-does-aging-affect-bipolar-disorder

Hamilton, Martin. n.d. "How to Control Mood Swings and Emotions." Accessed July 8, 2024. https://mindfulnessmethods.com/how-to-control-mood-swings-and-emotions/

Harvard Health Publishing. 2022. "Six Relaxation Techniques to Reduce Stress." Published February 2, 2022. https://www.health.harvard.edu/mind-and-mood/six-relaxation-techniques-to-reduce-stress

Henter, Ioline D., Lawrence T. Park, and Carlos A. Zarate. 2021. "Novel Glutamatergic Modulators for the Treatment of Mood Disorders: Current Status." *CNS Drugs* 35 (5): 527–43. doi:10.1007/s40263-021-00816-x.

Hicks, Joy. 2024. "12 Points in a Patient's Bill of Rights." Last modified February 24, 2024. https://www.verywellhealth.com/patient-bill-of-rights-2317484

Hoy, Toni. n.d. "Support Groups: Types, Benefits, and What to Expect." Accessed July 7, 2024. https://www.helpguide.org/articles/therapy-medication/support-groups.htm

IDCC Health Services. 2023. "How to Prepare for Psychiatry Appointment." Published October 12, 2023. https://idcchealth.org/blogs/how-to-prepare-for-psychiatry-appointment/

Indeed. 2023. "12 Strategies for Staying Focused on Your Goal (Plus Tips)." Last modified February 3, 2023. https://www.indeed.com/career-advice/career-development/focus-on-your-goal

International Bipolar Foundation. n.d. "11 Ways to Support Someone During Mania." Accessed July 6, 2024. https://ibpf.org/articles/11-ways-to-support-someone-during-mania/

International Bipolar Foundation. n.d. "Finding the Right Medication." Accessed July 5, 2024. https://ibpf.org/articles/finding-the-right-medication/

Jarrold, Jenna. 2023. "Family Focused Therapy." Last modified February 7, 2023. https://www.therapytribe.com/therapy/what-is-family-focused-therapy/

Jensen, Kate. 2023. "7 Tips to Explain a Bipolar Diagnosis to Your Child." Published June 30, 2023. https://www.healthline.com/health/bipolar-disorder/explaining-to-kids

Keener, Matthew T., and Mary L. Phillips. 2007. "Neuroimaging in Bipolar Disorder: A Critical Review of Current Findings." *Current Psychiatry Reports* 9 (6): 512–20. https://www.ncbi.nlm.nih.gov/pmc/articles/PMC2686113/.

Klein-Baer, Rosa. n.d. "How to Model Healthy Coping Skills." Accessed July 7, 2024. https://childmind.org/article/how-to-model-healthy-coping-skills/

Kohshour, Mojtaba Oraki, Sergi Papiol, Christopher R. K. Ching, and Thomas G. Schulze. 2022. "Genomic and Neuroimaging Approaches to Bipolar Disorder." *BJPsych Open* 8 (2): e36. doi:10.1192/bjo.2021.1082.

Krans, Brian. 2024. "Foods to Eat and Avoid with Bipolar Disorder." Last modified May 30, 2024. https://www.healthline.com/health/bipolar-disorder/foods-for-mania-and-depression

Kurczewska-Michalak, M., P. Lewek, B. Jankowska-Polańska, A. Giardini, N. Granata, M. Maffoni, E. Costa, L. Midão, and P. Kardas. 2021. "Polypharmacy

Management in the Older Adults: A Scoping Review of Available Interventions." *Frontiers in Pharmacology* 12 (November): 734045. doi:10.3389/fphar.2021.734045.

Lamoreux, Karen. 2021. "The 11 Best Mindfulness Books of 2022." Last modified December 21, 2021. https://psychcentral.com/health/best-mindfulness-books#_noHeaderPrefixedContent

Landmark. 2020. "The Benefits of More Informed Patients." Published April 7, 2020. https://www.landmarkhealth.org/resource/the-benefits-of-more-informed-patients/

Lebow, Hilary. 2022. "How to Prevent a Bipolar Episode." Last modified July 22, 2022. https://psychcentral.com/bipolar/prevention-of-bipolar-disorder

Lee, Janet and Karen Swartz. n.d. "Bipolar I Disorder." Accessed July 2, 2024. https://www.hopkinsguides.com/hopkins/view/Johns_Hopkins_Psychiatry_Guide/787045/all/Bipolar_I_Disorder

Leonard, Jayne. 2020. "What to Know About Telepsychiatry." Published April 20, 2020. https://www.medicalnewstoday.com/articles/telepsychiatry#what-is-it

MacMillan, Amanda. 2022. "How to Deal with Side Effects of Medication." Published November 14, 2022. https://www.webmd.com/a-to-z-guides/features/manage-drug-side-efects

Madeson, Melissa. 2024. "Holistic Therapy: Healing Mind, Body, and Spirit." Published February 23, 2024. https://positivepsychology.com/holistic-therapy/#different-types-of-holistic-therapy

Magellan Healthcare. 2020. "Best Practices for Behavioral Health Discharge Planning." Published December 2020. https://www.magellanofpa.com/documents/2021/07/best-practices-discharge-planning-sud-providers.pdf/

Martin, Elaina J. 2021. "How to Help a Loved One with Bipolar Disorder." Last modified March 24, 2021. https://psychcentral.com/blog/helping-your-partner-manage-bipolar-disorder

Martins, Julia. 2024. "18 Time Management Tips, Strategies, and Quick Wins to Get Your Best Work Done." Published February 12, 2024. https://asana.com/resources/time-management-tips

Maryville University. 2021. "The Importance of Celebrating Milestones." Published November 17, 2021. https://online.maryville.edu/blog/importance-of-celebrating-milestones/

Mayo Clinic. 2024. "A Holistic Approach to Integrative Medicine." Published June 4, 2024. https://mcpress.mayoclinic.org/living-well/a-holistic-approach-to-integrative-medicine/

Mayo Clinic. n.d. "Bipolar Disorder." Accessed July 2, 2024. https://www.mayoclinic.org/diseases-conditions/bipolar-disorder/diagnosis-treatment/drc-20355961

Mayo Clinic. n.d. "Seasonal Affective Disorder (SAD)." Accessed July 9, 2024. https://www.mayoclinic.org/diseases-conditions/seasonal-affective-disorder/diagnosis-treatment/drc-20364722

Mayo Clinic. n.d. "Sleep Aids: Understand Options Sold Without a Prescription." Accessed July 3, 2024. https://www.mayoclinic.org/healthy-lifestyle/adult-health/in-depth/sleep-aids/art-20047860

Mayo Clinic. n.d. "Stress Management." Accessed July 5, 2024. https://anxietycoach.mayoclinic.org/family-stress/stress-management-and-building-resilience/stress-management/

McMillen, Matt. 2021. "Why Structure is Everything with Bipolar Disorder." Last modified January 27, 2021. https://www.healthcentral.com/slideshow/structure-routine-important-with-bipolar

MedCircle. n.d. "Why is Mental Health Education Important?" Accessed July 10, 2024. https://medcircle.com/articles/mental-health-education/

Meissner, Morgan. 2024. "Answering Your Frequently Asked Questions About Antipsychotic Medication for Bipolar Disorder." Published February 14, 2024. https://www.medicalnewstoday.com/articles/antipsychotics-for-bipolar-disorder-faqs

Meissner, Morgan. 2021. "Managing the Side Effects of Bipolar Disorder Medication." Published July 7, 2021. https://psychcentral.com/bipolar/how-to-deal-with-common-side-effects-of-bipolar-medication

Melemis, Steven M. 2015. "Relapse Prevention and the Five Rules of Recovery." *The Yale Journal of Biology and Medicine* 88 (3): 325–32. https://www.ncbi.nlm.nih.gov/pmc/articles/PMC4553654/.

Mental Health America. n.d. "Time to Talk: Uncomfortable, but Important." Accessed July 6, 2024. https://mhanational.org/time-talk-uncomfortable-important

Mihajlovic, Stefan. 2024. "The Benefits and Importance of a Support System – A Care Guide for Self-Care and Success." Published February 28, 2024. https://www.mentalhealthcenter.org/benefits-and-importance-of-support-system/

Miller, Kori D. 2019. "What is Meditation Therapy and What are the Benefits." Published August 22, 2019. https://positivepsychology.com/meditation-therapy/

Mind. n.d. "Managing Conversations About Mental Health." Accessed July 6, 2024. https://www.mind.org.uk/media-a/4842/blp-managing-conversations-around-mental-health_v2.pdf

Mind Tools. n.d. "Critical Thinking." Accessed July 10, 2024. https://www.mindtools.com/a3ixqae/critical-thinking

Mind Tools. n.d. "SMART Goals." Accessed July 8, 2024. https://www.mindtools.com/a4wo118/smart-goals

Modglin, Lindsay. 2023. "5 Best Mental Health Apps to Try in 2024." Last modified July 5, 2023. https://www.forbes.com/health/mind/best-mental-health-apps/

Moezzi, Melody. 2023. "Maintaining Financial Stability with Bipolar Disorder." Last modified October 26, 2023. https://www.bphope.com/maintaining-financial-stability-with-bipolar-disorder/

Moore, Marissa. 2022. "In Need of Bipolar Disorder Hospitalization? Here's What to Expect." Published June 7, 2022. https://psychcentral.com/bipolar/bipolar-disorder-hospitalization

Morales-Brown, Louse. 2023. "Bipolar Disorder and Sleeping Too Much." Last modified August 24, 2023. https://www.medicalnewstoday.com/articles/bipolar-sleeping-too-much

Mosunic, Chris. n.d. "How to Build a Daily Routine: 10 Habits for a Productive Day." Accessed July 3, 2024. https://blog.calm.com/blog/daily-routine

Muinos, Lacey. 2023. "Tips and Help for Being a Caretaker to Someone with Bipolar Disorder." Las modified July 25, 2023. https://psychcentral.com/bipolar/challenges-for-caregivers-of-bipolar-disorder#caregiving

Myers, Wyatt. 2020. "Why You Need a Bipolar Disorder Crisis Plan." Last modified February 5, 2020. https://www.healthgrades.com/right-care/bipolar-disorder/why-you-need-a-bipolar-disorder-crisis-plan

Nall, Rachel. 2022. "Antidepressants and Bipolar Disorder." Published October 5, 2022. https://www.healthline.com/health/bipolar-disorder/antidepressants

Nash, Jo. 2019. "What is Positive Self-Talk? (Incl. Examples)." Published September 26, 2019. https://positivepsychology.com/positive-self-talk/

National Institute of Mental Health. n.d. "Bipolar Disorder." Accessed July 2, 2024. https://www.nimh.nih.gov/health/statistics/bipolar-disorder

National Alliance on Mental Illness. n.d. "Understanding Health Insurance." Accessed July 9, 2024. https://www.nami.org/Your-Journey/Individuals-with-Mental-Illness/Understanding-Health-Insurance/

National Institute of Mental Health. 2024 "Bipolar Disorder." Accessed July 2, 2024. https://www.nimh.nih.gov/health/topics/bipolar-disorder

NeuroLaunch. 2023. 'Bipolar Awareness: Understanding and Supporting Individuals with Bipolar Disorder." Published October 4, 2023. https://neurolaunch.com/bipolar-awareness/

NeuroLaunch. 2023. "The Connection Between Bipolar Disorder and Hormones." Published October 4, 2023. https://neurolaunch.com/bipolar-and-hormones/

NeuroLaunch. 2023. "The Ultimate Guide to Bipolar Mood Charts: Tracking and Managing Your Mood." Published October 4, 2023. https://neurolaunch.com/bipolar-mood-chart/

Nguyen, Julie. 2021. "15 Types of Therapy to Know and How to Find the Best One for You." Published October 29, 2021. https://www.mindbodygreen.com/articles/types-of-therapy

Notebooks and Planners. 2023. "Honest Journaling: Don't Hold Back When Journaling for Yourself." Published November 7, 2023. https://notebooksandplanners.com/honest-journaling/

O'Bryan, Amanda. 2021. "How to Perform Body Scan Meditation: 3 Best Scripts." Published December 4, 2021. https://positivepsychology.com/body-scan-meditation/

Osser, David. 2022. "Drug-Drug Interactions in Patients with Bipolar Disorder." Published May 12, 2022. https://www.psychiatrictimes.com/view/drug-drug-interactions-in-patients-with-bipolar-disorder

Ostacher, Michael J. 2011. "Bipolar and Substance Use Disorder Comorbidity: Diagnostic and Treatment Considerations." *Focus* 9 (4): 428–34. doi:10.1176/foc.9.4.foc428.

P., Abigail. 2024. "Cultivating Trust: 8 Essential Components for Relationship Success." Published April 8, 2024. https://extension.usu.edu/hru/blog/building-trust-in-relationships-guide-to-lasting-connection

Pastore, Alexandra. 2024. "Behind the Tech: Oura Is Keeping the Pulse on Health for Every Body." Published January 11, 2024. https://www.cnet.com/health/medical/show-your-therapist-how-well-you-slept-with-new-oura-data-sharing-feature/

Pedersen, Traci. 2022. "All About Postpartum Bipolar Disorder." Last modified July 26, 2022. https://psychcentral.com/bipolar/depression-often-turns-to-bipolar-illness-after-childbirth

Pederson, Traci. 2021. "Is Bipolar Disorder Hereditary?" Published August 27, 2021. https://psychcentral.com/bipolar/is-bipolar-genetic-causes-and-risk-factors

Plata, Mariana. 2018. "The Power of Routine in Your Mental Health." Published October 4, 2018. https://www.psychologytoday.com/us/blog/the-gen-y-psy/201810/the-power-of-routines-in-your-mental-health

Pombo, Emmie. 2019. "Self-Help Techniques for Coping with Mental Illness." Published February 1, 2019. https://www.nami.org/advocate/self-help-techniques-for-coping-with-mental-illness/

Psychology Today. n.d. "Dialectical Behavior Therapy." Accessed July 5, 2024. https://www.psychologytoday.com/us/therapy-types/dialectical-behavior-therapy

Purse, Marcia. 2023. "How Sleep and Bipolar Disorder Interact." Last modified November 22, 2023. https://www.verywellmind.com/how-sleep-and-bipolar-disorder-interact-379019

Quinn, Patrick D., and Brian M. D'Onofrio. 2020. "Nature Versus Nurture☆." In

Encyclopedia of Infant and Early Childhood Development (Second Edition), edited by Janette B. Benson, 373–84. Oxford: Elsevier. doi:10.1016/B978-0-12-809324-5.21826-9.

Raff, Jennifer. n.d. "How to Read and Understand a Scientific Paper." Accessed July 10, 2024. https://arc.duke.edu/how-to-read-and-understand-a-scientific-paper-a-guide-for-non-scientists/

Rendall, Jessica. 2023. "Show Your Therapist How Well You Slept with New Oura Data-Sharing Feature." Published August 30, 2023. https://www.cnet.com/health/medical/show-your-therapist-how-well-you-slept-with-new-oura-data-sharing-feature/

Rice University, 2020. "Staying Current with the Latest Research." Published December 3, 2020. https://graduate.rice.edu/news/current-news/staying-current-latest-research

Richards, Veryan. 2018. "The Importance of Language in Mental Health Care." *The Lancet Psychiatry* 5 (6): 460–61. doi:10.1016/S2215-0366(18)30042-7.

Riopel, Leslie. 2019. "28 Best Meditation Techniques for Beginners to Learn." Published November 28, 2019. https://positivepsychology.com/meditation-techniques-beginners/

Russo Law Group, P.C. 2024. "Legal Guardianship for Adults with Serious Mental Illness." Published May 31, 2024. https://vjrussolaw.com/legal-guardianship-for-adults-with-serious-mental-illness/

Schulz, Richard, Jill Eden, Committee on Family Caregiving for Older Adults, Board on Health Care Services, Health and Medicine Division, and Engineering National Academies of Sciences. 2016. "Family Caregiving Roles and Impacts." In *Families Caring for an Aging America*. National Academies Press (US). https://www.ncbi.nlm.nih.gov/books/NBK396398/.

Seven, Zuva. 2023. "Should You Tell Your Boss If You Have a Mental Health Condition." Last modified February 15, 2023. https://www.verywellmind.com/disclosing-a-mental-health-condition-5222448

Stanborough, Rebecca Joy. 2022. "Living with Bipolar 2 Disorder." Published June 23, 2022. https://psychcentral.com/bipolar/living-with-bipolar-disorder

Substance Abuse and Mental Health Services Administration. 2019. "Living with Bipolar Disorder: How Family and Friends Can Help." Published April 26, 2019. https://www.samhsa.gov/blog/living-bipolar-disorder-how-family-friends-can-help

Substance Abuse and Mental Health Services Administration. n.d. "Protection & Advocacy for Individuals (PAIMI) Program." Accessed July 10, 2024. https://www.samhsa.gov/paimi-program

Suni, Eric. 2023. "How to Fix Your Sleep Schedule." Last modified December 8,

2023. https://www.sleepfoundation.org/sleep-hygiene/how-to-reset-your-sleep-routine

Sutton, Jeremy. 2024. "18 Effective Thought-Stopping Techniques (& 10 PDFS)." Published February 2, 2024. https://positivepsychology.com/thought-stopping-techniques/

Swingle, Chris. 2024. "7 Tips from Financial Planners to Protect Your Money from Mania." Last modified May 21, 2024. https://www.bphope.com/bipolar-buzz/7-tips-from-financial-planners-to-protect-your-savings/

Tahmaseb-McConatha, Jasmin. 2021. "Creative Coping in Troubled Times." Published August 22, 2021. https://www.psychologytoday.com/us/blog/live-long-and-prosper/202108/creative-coping-in-troubled-times

Tartakovsky, Margarita. 2021. "Living with Bipolar Disorder: What to Expect." Last modified March 16, 2021. https://psychcentral.com/bipolar/living-with-bipolar-disorder

Turner, Joshua. 2023. "Pack Like a Pro: What to Bring for Inpatient Mental Health Treatment." Published September 5, 2023. https://aspireatlas.com/what-to-pack-for-inpatient-mental-health-treatment

University of Washington. n.d. "FAQ: How do I Know if My Sources are Credible/Reliable?" Accessed July 10, 2024. https://guides.lib.uw.edu/research/faq/reliable

U.S. Department of Education. n.d. "Disability Rights." Accessed July 9, 2024. https://www.ed.gov/coronavirus/factsheets/disability-rights

U.S. Equal Employment Opportunity Commission. n.d. "Depression, PTSD, and Other Mental Health Conditions in the Workplace: Your Legal Rights." Accessed July 7, 2024. https://www.eeoc.gov/laws/guidance/depression-ptsd-other-mental-health-conditions-workplace-your-legal-rights

U.S. Food and Drug Administration. 2022. "Finding and Learning about Side Effects (Adverse Reactions)," Last modified August 8, 2022. https://www.fda.gov/drugs/find-information-about-drug/finding-and-learning-about-side-effects-adverse-reactions

Vanbuskirk, Sarah. 2023. "What is Light Therapy and is it Right for You?" Last modified December 4, 2023. https://www.verywellmind.com/what-is-light-therapy-and-is-it-right-for-you-5097392

Vann, Madeline R. 2023. "The 10 Most Common Triggers for Bipolar Mood Episodes." Last modified January 12, 2023. https://www.everydayhealth.com/bipolar-disorder-pictures/biggest-triggers-of-bipolar-mood-swings.aspx

Verdolin, Jennifer. 2019. "3 Ways to Improve Cognitive Flexibility." Published December 3, 2019. https://www.psychologytoday.com/us/blog/wild-connections/201912/3-ways-improve-your-cognitive-flexibility

Wagner, Vivian. 2017. "The Magic of Freewriting." Published August 1, 2017.

https://www.psychologytoday.com/us/blog/the-creative-life/201708/the-magic-of-freewriting

Wells, Diana. 2019. "How Can Exercise Help Bipolar Disorder?" Last modified December 6, 2019. https://www.healthline.com/health/bipolar-disorder/exercise

Werner, Carly. 2023. "10 Tips for How to Advocate for Yourself at the Doctor." Published September 7, 2023. https://www.healthline.com/health/how-to-advocate-for-yourself-at-the-doctor

Wisner, Wendy. 2023. "The Link Between Hormones and Mental Health." Last modified June 5, 2023. https://www.verywellmind.com/the-link-between-hormones-and-mental-health-7500077

World Health Organization. 2021. "6 Ways to Take Care of Your Mental Health and Well-Being this World Mental Health Day." Published October 7, 2021. https://www.who.int/westernpacific/about/how-we-work/pacific-support/news/detail/07-10-2021-6-ways-to-take-care-of-your-mental-health-and-well-being-this-world-mental-health-day

Wright, Stephanie. 2021. "Tips for Dealing with Triggers in Recovery from Substance Use Disorders." https://psychcentral.com/addictions/5-tips-for-managing-triggers-during-addiction-recovery

Zrpath Behavioral Health Services. 2023. "The Power of Consistency in Behavioral Health: Your Path to Progress." Published October 31, 2023. https://www.linkedin.com/pulse/power-consistency-behavioral-health-your-path-progress-zarephath-iuxgc?trk=public_post_feed-article-content